Soulful Scripts:
Meditations, Inspirations, *and* Breathwork

for Yoga Teachers and Wellness Guides

Kelli Russell

ISBN: 978-1-7353492-3-7 (paperback)
ISBN: 978-1-7353492-4-4 (ebook)

Printed in the United States of America
First Printing - December, 2023

Published by Radical Enlightenment, LLC
radicalenlightenment.com

Dedication

I dedicate this book to my husband Kevin Russell, who provided for us so that I could be a stay-at-home mom for our daughter during her younger years and for supporting my yoga teaching, always. I am continually awestruck and thankful for all of your talents and gifts, all that you share, the amazing life partner that you are, and every hat that you wear. I am so grateful. I love you, babe!

To our daughter, Ryan Russell. You are the most beautiful, magical being I have ever met. I love you more than all of the universes boomeranged through infinity. Thank you for being you and showing me how to more fully accept all others without judgment. What a beautiful teacher you are.

To my wonderful mom Tricia Harris who taught me from an early age that I could be whatever I wanted to be in life (including encouraging me to be a drummer in a band, a tennis pro, a golf pro, a newscaster on TV, or a world traveler! haha!) and my dad Dave Harris who showed me that you can totally transform your life (he started running, eating healthy, and became a track coach after having open heart surgery in his late 40s) and always told me he was proud of me, whatever I did.

To Ann and Dan Russell, my second parents, for all of your love and support throughout the years in a multitude of ways.

To my yoga teachers, Selena Forman, who showed me what yoga could be (because of you, I fell in love with it), and Rached Maalouf, the closest thing to my Guru, who walked the walk and talked the talk.

And to all of the amazing students I've had the honor of guiding and practicing with throughout the years and the heartfelt relationships we've made. Connecting before and after class is my favorite part, and you are the reason that I love teaching.

Contents

Mini Meditations
(1-5 Minutes)

Short Meditations
(5-10 Minutes)

Long Meditations
(10-35 Minutes)

Wisdom Bytes

Inspirations

(Contents cont.)

Breathing Practices

FREE GIFT!

I'm so excited you've chosen this book as your trusted resource for meditation, breathwork, and spiritual instruction. To make a profound impact on your students' journey to self-discovery, inner peace, and personal growth, it's not just about sharing knowledge; it's about authentically connecting and actively engaging them.

Student engagement is the secret sauce that turns your classes into profound and transformative experiences.

As a token of my appreciation, here you'll find a treasure trove of strategies to boost student engagement and foster that vital connection.

Scan the QR CODE or **go to soulfulscripts.com** to get your free BONUS GIFT!

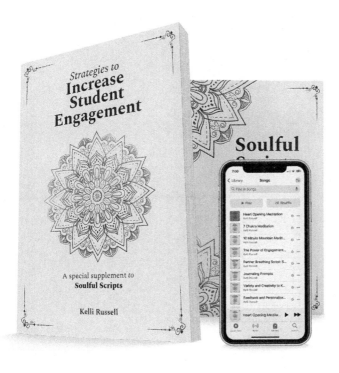

- **Strategies to Increase Student Engagement E-Book & Audiobook**

- **An Exclusive Partner Breathwork Script**

- **Plus 3 Guided Meditation Audio Tracks!**

INTRODUCTION

Welcome, Yoga & Meditation Teachers and Wellness Guides,

Soulful Scripts: Meditations, Inspirations, and Breathwork is not just a book; it's a conversation across the mat - a collection of the best resources from my 14-year teaching journey designed to help you guide your students through a holistic transformation that nurtures body, mind, and spirit, and leads them back to their authentic selves.

We've all been there—scrambling for that spark of inspiration just before a class or sifting through endless scraps of paper and digital notes. This book puts everything you need in one place, offering a structured, easy-to-follow format.

Think of this book as your trusted teacher's companion. It's here to save you time— time you'd rather spend connecting with your students, being present with your family, laughing with friends, or just soaking in the beauty of life.

Whether you need a quick quote to kick things off or an in-depth guided meditation, you're covered. And with the book divided into six user-friendly sections, you can easily pinpoint exactly what you need to complement the day's lesson:

1. Mini Meditations

2. Short Meditations

3. Long Meditations

4. Small Byte Inspirations

5. Inspirations

6. Breathing Practices

This book is here to help you:

- Handpick inspiring thoughts or messages for your class without the hassle

- Integrate specific breathing techniques that align with your session's goals

- Seamlessly conduct meditations of any duration, with ready-made scripts

- Create memorable, transformative experiences that keep your students returning

I'm so excited for you to start this journey with Soulful Scripts, for the difference it will make for you and your students, and for the moments of deep inner growth and freedom that will unfold within the magical experiences you offer.

Meditation doesn't change you into someone better than you were before.

Instead, it removes those things that shroud your highest self.

MEDITATIONS

HOW TO UTILIZE THESE MEDITATIONS

These meditations were created with yoga, meditation, and spiritual instructors in mind. Within these pages, you'll find meditation scripts as well as inspirational musings that can be read in yoga classes, meditation classes, and spiritual or self-development courses. *The italicized sentences are notes for the instructor :) If you want to share some of the background information found in the teacher's notes with your students, feel free!* Take your time reading the meditations with a relaxed rhythm and tone. Allow space for the words to settle in, and pause between each paragraph, as these in-between places can often be the most important and impactful part of the journey.

MEDITATION POSTURE

Meditation may have the greatest effects while seated, as the erect spine alerts the body and brain that it's time to pay attention, whereas a supine position may signify to the body and mind that it's time to sleep. However, for some individuals, a seated posture may cause strain or pain. Offer your students or group the option to lean back against a chair or a wall, or even to lie down.

Guide postural alignment, whether seated or supine, before each and every meditation. Remind your students that each time they sit for meditation, it's beneficial to switch the crossing of the legs, changing which leg goes in front. This way, over time there will be more balanced flexibility in the hips, knees, ankles, feet, and really, the entire body.

If the following props are available, suggest that they sit on a folded-up blanket, bolster, or meditation pillow for greater comfort.

Optimal Seated Posture:
Guide lifting the sternum (breastbone), drawing the shoulder blades down the back, relaxing the hip flexors, and gently engaging the stomach muscles to support the spine.

There are a few meditations that are best experienced lying down. This will be stated within the italicized teacher's notes.

Optimal Supine (Lying Down) Position:
Invite students to place a bolster or pillow underneath their knees (if available) or place their feet a little wider than hip's width apart, allowing their toes to flop out. Guide them to lengthen their spine, tuck their shoulder blades under, placing arms out by sides, palms facing up, allowing their chest to open.

GUIDING THEM OUT

At the end of each meditation, guide taking some deeper breaths, bringing awareness to their bodies, opening their eyes, and shifting posture (such as from lying down to seated) in the way that makes the most sense for you and the structure of your class or offering. Coming back to seated, remind them to lengthen their spines and lift their chests.

For some meditations, I've included post-meditation insights and suggestions for students to bridge the practice into their lives. You may wish to read these when students still have their eyes closed so that they can receive the information while in the meditative state, then have them open their eyes. If you are guiding a lying down meditation or savasana, decide if it makes more sense to have practitioners receive the information while lying down with their eyes closed or after they return to a seated posture.

WHY MEDITATE

The brain spends most of its time looping - replaying the past, worrying about the future, planning, and avoiding pain. Its primary job is to keep us safe.

At first, when we sit or lie down, we notice it even more. But the point is not to sit still, completely devoid of thoughts. This is impossible! For the moment we realize, *"I am so deep in meditation that I have merged with the universe!"*, it's a thought!

The point really is to FALL AWAKE. We simply notice whatever shows up, allow it to morph, shift, dissolve...all so that we can be aware of what is present. We notice and release our attraction and aversion to things. We see the tricks of the mind: the distractor, the bully, the judge.

Sometimes feelings come up that we've been avoiding. But there is suddenly space for it all. There is space for everything. And then we start to experience what is beyond all of that. We realize that we are the serene PRESENCE observing it all.

This heightened presence then overflows into our daily lives while we eat, when we engage with others, when we love, and when we work.

We have awakened.

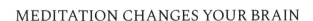

MEDITATION CHANGES YOUR BRAIN

Research shows that what you focus on, you will get: If you focus on your breath or a mantra during meditation, your brain will restructure itself to make concentration easier.

If you focus on a state of calmness, your brain will be more resilient to stress. If you meditate on love and acceptance, your brain will receive and send out signals that allow you to feel more connected to others.

Meditators have more gray matter in brain regions associated with attention, emotional regulation, and emotional flexibility.

MINI MEDITATIONS
(1-5 minutes)

These mini meditations are short and sweet.

They can be utilized at the end of a yoga class during the first part of savasana, or to start or end a class, spiritual event, or activity.

Guide body posture first, as appropriate for either sitting or lying down.

They are all between one and five minutes, but you could add more time for silence before opening eyes if you wish to lengthen them.

Choose the mini meditation (the title says it all) that makes the most congruent sense for what you'll be focused on, or have focused on throughout the practice.

RELAXING

Close your eyes.

Relax your shoulders.

Soften your neck.

Relax your jaw and your cheeks.

Relax your tongue in your mouth.

Soften your eyelids, your eyebrows, and the space between them. Soften your forehead.

Relax your scalp and ears.

Allow this feeling of relaxation to flow down into your body like honey.

Flowing gently downwards through your arms, your chest, into your abdomen, your pelvis, thighs, lower legs, and feet.

Feel this feeling of relaxation throughout your entire being.

Wait a minute.

When you are ready...gently open your eyes.

MAGICAL ERASING BRUSH

Close your eyes. Imagine a magical brush with long, soft bristles. Instead of painting, this brush erases.

Starting at your toes and feet this brush goes back and forth, back and forth, erasing them. Erasing ankles, shins, knees, and upper thighs. Back and forth, back and forth.

Erasing hips and pelvis, hands, arms, and torso. Erasing your neck and jaw, tongue, nose, ears, and eyes. All your senses. Back and forth, back and forth.

Your brain is the last thing to go. The voice in your head, all of your thoughts and memories, gone. There is no longer a physical membrane between yourself and the universe. No longer a boundary.

You are part of the energy of the universe. You can see, but not with your eyes. And you can hear, but not with your ears. You know, but not with your brain. You are simply BEING.

Feeling the flow of the energy of the universe for the next ___ minutes. *(As long as you've allotted for this meditation)*

(When it's time to complete the meditation) Allow your body to materialize slowly, cells gaining structure, heart beating, blood flowing.

Take a few deep breaths into your lungs.

Welcome back. Slowly open your eyes.

PEACE EXPANDING

Close your eyes.

Draw the feeling of peace into your body. If it's hard to find it, remember a time when you felt it before, or imagine what it would feel like.

Once you sense it, notice where in your body you feel it the most. Localize it.

What does it feel like? Send the feeling outwards now to encompass your entire body. Expand it out farther, beyond your body into the space you inhabit.

Intensify the feeling, then expand it out even farther, encompassing your neighborhood. Throughout the city.

Wider, throughout the state... the country...the continent...then throughout our entire world.

Feeling Peace. Being Peace. (*Wait a minute or two*)

When you're ready...open your eyes.

LIFE VISUALIZING

Close your eyes.

Sometimes it seems like it takes a long time to bring your hopes and dreams to life. In the quantum field, it only takes an instant.

Let's jump two years into the future, seeing the things that you want to experience happening in your life.

Visualize yourself doing work that you love, experiencing success in whatever way is meaningful to you..., seeing your romantic life flourishing..., enjoying time with friends..., with family..., seeing yourself contributing to others in some way..., and enjoying some time in solitude.

Seeing your body looking healthy and vibrant.

How do you feel?

By seeing yourself and your life in this way, feeling the feelings of it, the same chemicals are released as if you actually did those things.

This makes it easier for these things to come to fruition. You have created a road map. Your system says, "Oh! That's what you want? Okay then!"

Slowly open your eyes.

GRATITUDE

Close your eyes.

Consider the past 24 hours and think of as many things as you can to feel appreciation for. If you can't think of many things within the last day, span out and consider the past week.

They might be little pleasures like your bed and soft pillows, your morning coffee or tea, or the rain that came down last night.

Look at what happened at home and at work *(if it applies)*, while running errands, during your free time, with family members, friends, and pets.

Big or small, remember them all.

(Allow a minute or two to contemplate.)

Notice what it feels like in your body and mind now.

It is impossible to hold fear, anxiety, and worry at the same time as gratitude and appreciation.

Remember that you can do this mini-meditation anytime you find yourself downward-spiraling, to shift yourself into a higher state.

Gently open your eyes.

FORGIVING

Close your eyes.

Bring to mind someone you're harboring negative thoughts or feelings about.

If no one comes to mind, perhaps there's someone from your past. Picture them standing in front of you.

When we hold on to negative thoughts and feelings, it is us that we continue to harm, not them.

And it keeps what happened active in our field.

If you would like to release it, bring awareness to your heart, guiding a feeling of warmth and peace there.

In your mental landscape say, "I forgive and release you. And for any harm I've done, even if just for holding onto negative thoughts or feelings, please forgive and release me".

Picture their eyes and face softening knowing that their heart has received your message.

The image in your mind clears.

A weight has been lifted.

You feel lighter, freer, better.

When you are ready, open your eyes.

RESTORE

Close your eyes.

Take a deep, full, rich breath in, and exhale letting it all go.

Release control of your breath.

Relax everything.

Every muscle, every tissue.

Feel a sense of deep relaxation settling in.

Your body is healing and restoring as you rest in stillness.

Just be here now, resting and restoring, healing and rejuvenating.

Wait a minute or two.

When you are ready...open your eyes.

WINDY THOUGHTS

Have you ever been in a windy place? At first, you hear the howling wind as it moves around objects.

Almost like the sound of the ocean. It ebbs and flows. Whooshes.

After a while, you tune it out. It moves into the background.

Can you allow your thoughts to be like the wind?

Can you allow them to drift into the background?

There's a noticing, then a letting go.

Once this state is found, you are meditating.

THE SUSPENDED SPACE OF NOW

Close your eyes.

You have everything you need in this moment.

Relax your body. Clear your mind.

Allow yourself to float in the suspended space of now.

(Wait a minute or two)

When you are ready, open your eyes

PRESENCE

Close your eyes.

Feel the sense of your own BEING-ness.

Your inner radiance.

Pure consciousness.

Feel the expanded state of stillness here.

Feel the pure presence that you just cultivated.

Wait a minute or two.

When you are ready, open your eyes.

POSSIBILITIES

Close your eyes. It's time to release.

Release control of your breath. Relax everything.

Every muscle, every tissue. Feel how in tune you are with your body. Feel the state of calmness and clarity you have cultivated.

In this space, possibilities are limitless. Reside in this space for the next few minutes.

Wait for 2-3 minutes. When you are ready, open your eyes.

STRESS RELEASE

Close your eyes.

Take a full, deep breath through your nose from the bottom to the top of your lungs, and hold your breath at the top.

Notice any stress building up as you hold it.

When you're ready, let it all go with a powerful exhale through your mouth.

Again, inhale, fill up your stomach then your chest and as you hold your breath at the top, see if there's any stress or tension.

When you're ready, exhale with a strong sigh, releasing all of it.

One last time, take a slow, deep breath and fill up all the little spaces that you can.

Exhale, and let it all go.

Allow your breath to normalize as you feel a deep stillness wash over you.

Anchor yourself in the present and know that everything is unfolding in your life with perfect timing.

When you are ready,

Open your eyes.

MENTAL VACATION

Bring your spine into long, straight alignment.

Close your eyes.

Imagine that you're sitting down in the middle of the most beautiful place.

It may be a beach, a meadow, or on top of a mountain ridge. Whatever place is the most peaceful for you.

Sitting here, look around in your mental landscape at all the beauty surrounding you.

Notice the smell and the way the air feels on your skin.

Allow more details to fill in.

Maybe sounds, animals, flowers...you feel so relaxed here. So content.

The feeling remains with you as the image begins to dissolve.

Know that you can visit whenever you want.

Take some slow, deep breaths

and gently open your eyes.

LIGHT BEAM

Close your eyes.

Imagine yourself totally encompassed within a beam of shimmery, bright light. This light is a high frequency that releases any pent-up emotions. It dissipates anything heavy or dense you've been carrying with you. Here there is infinite wisdom, infinite consciousness.

Allow yourself to bask in this light for the next couple of minutes.

Wait 2 minutes

You feel different now that all heaviness has lifted.

Light...*(wait a few moments)*,

open...*(wait a few moments)*,

expansive...*(wait a few moments)*,

and free.

Wait a minute.

These qualities remain with you as you open your eyes.

ALLOWING

Close your eyes. Allow your breath, feelings, and all sensations to be exactly as they are.

Allow whatever thoughts that are present to be there.

Observe and witness the spacious presence of awareness.

Being spacious presence.

Pure awareness.

When you're ready, keep this new state of awareness with you, and gently open your eyes.

REJUVENATION

Close your eyes. Notice the tingly aliveness of every cell in your body.

Experience the magic of your own physiology.

The vibration of health rejuvenating any areas that need it,

bringing your system to perfect harmony.

Tingly and alive, healthy and vibrant.

When you're ready, softly open your eyes.

BEING

Close your eyes.

Without trying to change it in any way, just observe your breath.

Be here with whatever comes up without judging it in any way.

Simply experience whatever you're experiencing.

If your mind starts to go too far down a thought path,

notice your body and your breathing again.

Find yourself just simply being.

Nowhere to go,

just being completely present.

Wait for a minute or two.

When you're ready,

softly open your eyes.

ENERGY AMPLIFIER

Close your eyes and take a few deep breaths.

If you feel tired, depleted, or apathetic, remember that you have access to the field of energy at all times.

You are living within a grid of energy.

The energy of all that is.

The energy that creates worlds.

It is all around you.

You are literally bathing in it.

Visualize opening up your crown chakra and drawing vibrant energy in through the crown of your head,

filling you up until you sense that you are completely full of pure energy,

pure love,

and pure light.

Like turning up a dial,

you can almost hear it.

"Mmmmmmmmmmmmmm"

SHORT MEDITATIONS
(5-10 minutes)

These meditations are 5-10 minutes long.
Some can be lengthened to any amount of time.

BREATH SENSATION MEDITATION

Time: 5 minutes to as long as you like

Teacher's Note:

Breath-focused meditations are great for beginners to advanced meditators. The breath is one of the easiest anchors to tune into because there is a continuous rhythm, however, training the brain to remain focused on it can take a lot of consistent practice.

You can choose to spend the first half of the meditation focusing on belly breathing, and the second half focusing on nostril breathing or can select only one for the entire time.

Today we'll be practicing a breath sensation meditation.

This is one of those practices that takes a moment to learn but a lifetime to master. Let's start our journey into mastery now ;)

We'll start with Belly Breathing.

Begin by noticing your breath.

Inhale through your nose, and exhale through your nose.

If you find that you're breathing primarily from your chest, then guide your breath lower, into your belly.

Practice a few rounds until it starts to feel more comfortable.

(Wait for a few rounds of breath)

Now that you've got the hang of it, begin to observe the sensation of your belly rising and falling with the occurrence of your breath.

Feel, as you inhale, your belly extending, and feel, as you exhale, your belly softening.

Continue to focus on the rise and fall of your stomach as you inhale and exhale.

If at any time your mind wanders to something else, notice that it's happened, then with compassion, tether it back to feeling and noticing the sensation of the rise and fall of your belly as you breathe.

Keep your awareness connected to your breath in this way for the next ____ *(the amount of time allotted)* minutes.

Next, we'll move into Nostril Breathing.

Begin to notice the subtle sensation of your breath as it enters and exits your nostrils with your lips sealed.

Keep in mind that you are not manipulating your breath in any way, but rather noticing what's happening.

You might discover that when the air goes into your nose it's a little cooler, and once warmed through your system, it feels a little warmer as you exhale.

Stay connected to the sensation of the air going into and out of your nostrils.

If your mind wanders, notice that it's happened, then gently guide yourself back to the sensation of the air going in and out of your nose.

There is no judgment if your mind drifts, just notice that it has drifted, and come back to the sensation of the air going in and out of your nose.

Continue to observe the sensation of your breath in this way for the next _____ *(the amount of time allotted)* minutes.

GUIDING THEM OUT

*Read this part only **if you guided both the belly and nostril breathing**:*
Tune in to the sound of my voice.

Notice if it was easier for you to stay focused on the belly breathing or the nostril breathing.

What feelings did each elicit within you?

*Read this part **if you only guided one**:*
Tune into the sound of my voice.

What feelings did this breathing meditation elicit within you as you practiced?

How do you feel now?

There is no right or wrong answer.

SILENT MANTRA MEDITATIONS

Time: 5 minutes, to as long as you like

Teacher's Note:

A silent mantra is a word or sentence repeated over and over in order to train mental focus and create a conscious and subconscious resonance (if in the theta brain-wave state) with what is being said.

You can either guide only one mantra that you pre-select, or you can list the options out loud and let your students decide which one they would personally like to use, with the additional option of creating their own.

The Script:

A silent mantra is a great way to focus a busy mind toward a desired state of being. Our minds tend to think about 80% negative thoughts, so this practice can help ingrain a new positive thought.

I will offer some ideas. You can choose one of these, or create your own. Select the one that provides the most benefit for you right now.

Infinite possibilities surround me now

Letting go, letting be

My life is unfolding in perfect timing

My body returns to the blueprint of health

I give and receive love freely

Repeat each one again

Or remember, you can create one of your own.

Once you have selected your mantra,

close your eyes,

and say it over and over silently in your mind at a nice, slow, rhythmic pace

for the next _____ minutes.
(the time that you've allotted for this meditation)

If your mind wanders to something else, no worries, just bring it back to your mantra and continue to repeat it.

GUIDING THEM OUT

Release the words now.

Start to take some slow, deep breaths and feel your body.

Notice the resonance, the aftereffect of this meditation.

Bring your hands to your breastbone in prayer position.

Bow in, chin to chest to honor this practice, the power of your mantra, and its ability to redirect your thoughts, and thus, your reality.

OBJECT FOCUSED MEDITATION

Time: 5 minutes to as long as you'd like

Teacher's Note:

When I was learning to meditate, I found this one to be fun and easy. Our group practiced with a white candle. It was cool to see the color variant of the flame and how the smoke danced as I gazed. After staring at it for several minutes, once I closed my eyes, I could recreate the image in my mind.

There are two ways that you can practice this meditation: either imagining an object (without the physical item in front of you) or using an actual object.

If you're using an actual object, you can bring a crystal, a pencil, a lit candle (make sure this is safe with a plate or something underneath it), a water bottle, or anything that you wish. Find something fairly simple. If you're guiding a group, you can have them sit in a circle, and place a single item in the middle of the group. You could also have smaller groups each circled around an item, or you can bring enough items for each practitioner to have their own to gaze at. You may even ask your students ahead of time to bring their own.

Decide if you are guiding option 1 (imagining an object in your mind's eye) or option 2 (utilizing a physical object), and only guide that one.

This meditation is an attention training and visualization exercise that enhances your ability to remain alert and focused. It's best done while seated, with a tall spine. Feel free to place a bolster, block, or pillow underneath your hips for support.

Option 1: IMAGINING AN OBJECT IN YOUR MIND'S EYE

Select an object, either real or imagined, to visualize.

You'll be staying with this particular object for the entire meditation.

It can be any object of your choosing.

Some ideas for objects to focus on are something simple like an apple or pear, a lotus flower, or even a purple moon from another galaxy.

Something you would find interesting to meditate on for a while.

Close your eyes and bring to life an image of this object within your mental landscape.

As you see it in your mind, begin adding more and more details to it.

The color or colors become crisper.

Notice the texture that it appears to have.

For the next ____ minutes *(the time you've allotted for this meditation)*, bring as much rich detail to the object as you can,

and stay connected to "seeing" it for as long as you can.

If your mind wanders off to something else,

just simply bring it back to visualizing the object.

Option 2: UTILIZING A PHYSICAL OBJECT

For this meditation, you will place an actual object in front of the meditator(s). Here's an example of how you could utilize a candle for this purpose:

Place a candle in front of you and light it. *(Make sure it's safe - either on a large plate or within a candle holder of some sort, as you'll be closing your eyes and you don't want anything to catch fire).*

Gaze at the color of the wax.

Is it all one color, or are there color gradients?

See the shape, and notice the circumference.

Bring your awareness to the wick.

How long is it?

What kind of flame does this candle produce?

Does the air cause the flame to dance around or is it steady and somewhat still?

Notice the color of the flame.

The color at the flame's base, the main portion of the flame, and the very tip of the flame.

Now close your eyes, and call to mind as many details as you can.

See its shape, texture, and color.

See the flame. Recreate it.

Keep adding in finer and finer features.

Stay connected to the image of the candle within your mind for the duration of your meditation, *(let them know how long the meditation will be).*

If your mind wanders, bring it back to the mental image of the candle.

If you lose the mental image, you can always open your eyes and take a peek until you've got it again ;).

GUIDING THEM OUT

If you find yourself unable to sleep at night, practice visualizing this image again within your mind.

You may find that you drift off to sleep, but if you are still awake, instead of getting frustrated, you can use it as manifestation practice.

Once you get proficient at visualizing this image, then start imagining a scene of what you'd like to experience in your life.

A trip you want to take, an experience with a loved one, or doing something amazing with your work or creativity.

Add emotions and your other senses as you visualize for added power.

Seeing it serves as a rehearsal.

The experience is now more real to you, making it more likely that you create a similar experience in your waking life.

WITNESS MEDITATION

Time: 5 minutes to as long as you'd like

Teacher's Note:
This meditation is so powerful!

Training witness consciousness invites people to truly step into a state of enlightenment, becoming awake and aware as they observe feelings, sensations, and the mind's thinking.

It is then that they realize that they are not these things, they are the pure consciousness behind them.

Close your eyes. Take a few slow, deep breaths.

For this meditation, you will simply be the observer of your thoughts, feelings, and sensations as they move across your field of awareness.

Allow them to come and go. Look how they arrive, morph, and dissolve.

Practice being unattached to what you observe. Just watching.

It may go something like this, "I'm noticing that I feel a hunger pang... I see that I'm thinking about what happened with Lisa last week... I see that my mind is bringing up that work meeting that I have on Monday... I notice that my foot is falling asleep now...".

You are just witnessing all of it.

Watching it happen.

There may also be some gaps between thoughts and sensations where you are simply being.

Continue practicing this for the next ___minutes.
(the remaining time you've allotted for this meditation)

GUIDING THEM OUT

Begin to take some deep breaths into your belly.

As you observed the coming and going of thoughts, feelings, and emotions, you may have noticed that you had more of a pulled-back perspective.

That there was a deeper you witnessing what was happening. Pure consciousness.

As you re-enter your life, keep witnessing and observing.

Thoughts, emotions, and sensations (whether you deem them good or bad) change constantly.

The more you notice them, experience them, and allow them to flow through you, the less resistant you will be, and the more present you will become.

And the deeper truth that you realize is that YOU ARE the witness, the consciousness behind them all.

LIKE A TRAIN THROUGH A STATION

Time: 5 minutes

> *Teacher's Note:*
> *This meditation helps people become more awake and aware of their thinking without getting entangled by their thoughts.*
>
> *By becoming good at this, they will lessen stress, anxiety, worry, and depression by not going down the rabbit hole of limiting or negative thoughts.*
>
> *The thoughts begin to lose their power and practitioners maintain greater equanimity as they observe them.*

Have you ever become entangled in a sticky thought?

You start ruminating about something and go deeper and deeper down the rabbit hole.

This meditation helps you train your ability to disentangle yourself by becoming more awake and aware of your thoughts, consciously letting them drift by while maintaining equanimity.

Close your eyes, and relax your facial muscles.

Feel your eyebrows and forehead relax.

Your mouth and jaw soften as you notice your natural breath going in and out.

For this meditation, you will simply allow your thoughts to come and go, like trains passing through a station.

See yourself as the station, and the thoughts as the trains passing by.

Do not allow any train to get stuck in the station for too long.

If you find yourself getting stuck in a thought, just notice that it's happened, and then see the train leave the station.

Off it goes.

Continue this practice for the next ____minutes.
(the time you've allotted for this meditation)

GUIDING THEM OUT

Take a moment to recognize how you feel.

Did you find a lot of trains getting stuck or were they able to flow by pretty easily?

If you found them getting stuck, this is a practice you can continue.

By training your mind in this way, you begin to realize that thoughts are just coming and going and they start to lose their power over you.

This lessens stress, anxiety, worry, and depression.

You become more empowered, calm, and relaxed as you realize that you are not your thoughts.

LABELING THOUGHTS

Time: 5 minutes to as long as you'd like

Teacher's Note:

The notion that meditation is about clearing the mind of all thoughts has kept many people from trying meditation because they think it's impossible, and has caused many people to stop meditating because of how challenging it is.

Instead of stopping thoughts, especially in the early years of practicing meditation, I believe it is more accessible and valuable to offer meditations like these, where we just simply notice what is present.

This provides a point of focus for the meditator, increasing awareness, and they start to see the thoughts for what they are: just thoughts!

Some believe that while meditating, we must be devoid of thoughts.

However, the more we push thoughts away, the more resistance is created.

What we resist, persists.

When we attempt to push thoughts out of our minds, they tend to hide behind the curtains of our consciousness.

Still there, lurking.

When you identify a thought, though, and give it a name, you may find that it's little more than nothing.

It loses its power and disappears!

You can notice a thought, or become "lost in a thought."

Consider the difference. Becoming aware of a thought is like watching a movie, rather than being a character in the movie.

For this meditation, you will practice being the watcher, the observer.

Begin now. Close your eyes and just watch.

You may experience pockets of space without thoughts, but if any thoughts arise, assign a one-word label to them.

A present tense, active word with an -ing at the end.

For example, if you have a thought that you're hungry, assign the label "hungering".

If you're replaying a conversation that you had with someone, wondering if you handled it right, you could label it "worrying" or "ruminating".

If you are going over what you're going to do for the rest of the day, you could label it "planning".

You will notice that thoughts are coming and going.

Allow the thought to come.

Give it a label.

Watch it disappear.

Continue this for the next ___minutes.
(the time you've allotted for this meditation)

GUIDING THEM OUT

Now that you've experienced this meditation, apply this to your life.

Instead of trying to rid yourself of thoughts, (a nearly impossible task), become MORE aware of them.

Observe your thoughts and allow them to flow through you, without getting overpowered by them.

The more that you witness the coming and going of thoughts, the more you become conscious.

This is what it means to be awake, rather than sleepwalking through life.

With practice, you will maintain longer stretches of consciousness.

Instead of feeling like life is happening to you, you will be choosing your reactions, guiding your life.

DEEPER THAN THAT

Time: 5-7 minutes

Teacher's Note:

This meditation is all about releasing attachment to one's identity based on external qualifiers.

What happens if someone has fully identified themselves as a professional football player and they become injured in a way that ends their career?

This practice helps people recognize their innate value beneath their roles, jobs, and characteristics.

Depending on who you're guiding this meditation for, select the appropriate words based on who is present.

For example, if there are all women, there is no need to mention father, son, or brother.

Close your eyes, and for the next minute, simply notice the natural rise and fall of your breath and the natural rise and fall of your thought waves.

(Wait 1 minute)

Consider now, how you identify yourself:

mother, daughter, sister, father, son, brother, friend, employee, employer, tall, short, rich, poor, lucky, unlucky, introvert, extrovert.

Add any other descriptive words that you associate with.

What other bodily characteristics? What other personality traits?

What astrological sign or other things like that?

What job do you do at work or within your household?

(Wait about 30 seconds)

Many of these descriptors keep you boxed in, and unavailable for change.

Ask yourself, "What within me is deeper than these things?"

(Wait about 30 seconds to a minute)

"What is actually here now?"

(Wait about 30 seconds to a minute)

You might notice that your mind starts to quiet, and the mental debris starts to clear away.

"What is underneath this identity I'm so attached to?"

(Wait about 30 seconds to a minute)

"What is already whole and complete within me now?"

(Wait about 30 seconds to a minute)

You might notice that your heart starts to open and your body relaxes.

You are more aware, in this state of BEING-NESS.

This state of presence.

Your being-ness is right here.

Allow whatever is present to unfold.

(Provide 1-2 minutes for silence)

GUIDING THEM OUT

Bring your hands to prayer position at your heart.

As you leave this meditation, remember who you truly are, at the center of your core.

SPATIAL REFERENCING

Time: 3-8 minutes

Teacher's Note:
This meditation is great for helping to shift people out of stress and
anxiety quickly.

Noticing one's surroundings and experiencing oneself proprioceptively is
very grounding and calming to the nervous system.

This one is great to use at the beginning of your class, event, or meditation
group.

Let's get grounded and allow ourselves to come fully into the present moment by guiding ourselves into our bodies and sensing our relationship to our surroundings.

Begin by lengthening your spine.

Lift your chest and grow a bit taller from through the crown of your head.

Look down and to the right. See what you notice there.

What objects, colors, textures?

Now look to the lower left side. What do you see?

Scan the space in between.

In front of you.

Shift your gaze higher now, right up the center.

Notice what you see there.

Now look up and to the right. See what stands out.

What smaller details can you notice?

Look up and to the left and do the same. Any different shapes or colors?

Now to the center, but go higher with your eyes.

Scan the area directly above you, and then the whole field up above you, everything that you can take in.

Slowly turn your head to your right and look behind you.

Start at the ground level, then let your eyes travel higher, noticing what there is to notice on the way up.

Look all the way up.

Gently bring your head back to neutral, then turn your head to the left.

Starting at the ground, see what you can see.

Allow your eyes to travel slowly upwards, taking in what is behind you.

Let your eyes once again travel all the way up. Notice what is there.

Gently bring your head to face forward again.

Keeping your head facing forward, use a broad perspective and your peripheral vision to take in the whole picture now, the entirety.

Feel yourself where you are, in this time and place.

Notice where you are in relation to the other things around you.

Feel the earth beneath you.

Grounded and centered in your own body.

Check-in with yourself: How do you feel in this moment now?

GUIDING THEM OUT

Utilize this mini-meditation anytime throughout your day, anywhere.

Sitting, standing, or lying down.

It brings you into the present moment and grounds you.

If you feel unsafe or in fight or flight mode, it helps you get in touch with your surroundings so that your nervous system can calm down.

If you feel untethered, it helps guide you back into your body.

ASK YOUR BODY MEDITATION

Time: 5 to 10 minutes

Teacher's Note:
It's pretty wild - even though this is a body meditation, the inquiry led me through one of the most meaningful spiritual experiences I've had to date.

Our meditation group had done about 20 minutes of meditative binaural beats music followed by these questions, asked at a slow pace.

It felt like the answers I received came directly from my soul!

Feel free to include binaural beats music or a Solfeggio frequency of your choosing, and lengthen the meditation any amount that you wish.

Take several slow, deep, diaphragmatic breaths.

Now allow your breath to soften and normalize, and continue to notice your breath going in and out for the next couple of minutes.

Set the intention to put your highest self in charge now.

Your wisdom self, your superconscious.

Begin to scan your body for tension.

You may notice pain, tension, or simply that your awareness is drawn to a certain place in your body.

Once you've identified a specific place in your body, ask the pain or tension what its name is.

Wait 30 seconds.

Ask, "What are you here to tell me?"

Wait 60 seconds.

Ask if the name of the sensation is still the same now.

Ask, "What is your name now?"

Have a conversation.

Ask any questions you wish, listen for the answers, and ask follow-up questions until you experience understanding.

Allow them to continue for 2-3 minutes.

GUIDING THEM OUT

As we end the meditation, begin to breathe deeper.

If you received a message that provided insight that was meaningful for you, ask yourself if there are any action steps or adjustments to make in your life based on the information you received.

What are between 1-3 things that you could do right now? Things you would actually do.

Commit to follow through on your action steps, if you have any, in order to bring these positive changes into your life.

A WALK ON THE SAND

Time: 7-10 min

Teacher's Note:

While I was on vacation in Ocean City, NJ walking on the beach, I decided to really be present as I walked.

The beach was expansive, there was a cool breeze, and I saw the glitter of the sun's rays bouncing off of the surface of the ocean.

Hardly anyone else was out, and I seemed to be on this exploratory journey by myself.

What I kept getting drawn to, was the changing sensation of the sand's consistency beneath my feet. The journey unfolded as this walking meditation that I share with you here.

Imagine that you're at the beach, lying on a towel.

The air is just right, not too hot, not too cool.

The sun softly warms your skin.

See if you can smell the salty sea air. Hear the seagull as it passes by, and the sound of the ocean waves crashing against the shore.

In your mental landscape, you decide to slowly sit up and open your eyes.

You see the sun's reflection on the water and the glittery sea spray.

You decide to stand and go for a walk.

At first, you notice the sensation of crunchy sand underneath your feet as you walk parallel to the ocean.

As you look down, you see a myriad of tiny seashell particles throughout the sand.

You walk forward and feel the prickly pieces underneath your feet. You hear a crunchy sound with each step.

Wait 20 seconds.

Soon the sand softens to the texture of powdered sugar, pillowy underneath your footsteps.

What a difference. Luxurious, soft.

You continue for some time, feeling the mild sunlight on your chest and shoulders.

Wait 20 seconds.

The sand starts to become soggy and wet. Your feet sink down with each step, requiring more effort. Slogging through, you hear the sucking sound as you pull each foot up.

Wait 20 seconds.

Pretty soon the sand becomes firm-packed.

Drier, almost like concrete.

You feel taller as your feet remain completely on the surface.

You straighten your back and walk easier.

Wait 20 seconds.

As if by magic, up ahead you see your towel laid out on the sand.

You head over to it and decide to sit down.

You take one last glance at the beautiful ocean in front of you and the way the light sparkles on its surface and decide to lie down.

You realize that all this time you have been noticing, just noticing. Fully immersed in the present moment.

Your attention focused on your feet in the sand and the ever-changing sensations.

Some so soft and pillowy. Some uncomfortable and prickly.

But in the seat of the observer, you have been so calm and present.

Relaxed and easy as you experienced the variation.

You have been in a state of pure awareness.

Wait 20 seconds (or as long as you've allotted for this meditation).

GUIDING THEM OUT

Allow yourself to come back to this time and place now by slowly bringing your awareness back.

Lengthen your spine, and guide some deeper breaths into your lungs, expanding your belly as you breathe.

What if you could experience the ever-changing conditions of your life like this?

Some things we go through are easy and pleasant, and some are challenging or painful.

What if you remained in the seat of the observer, accepted what was happening, and felt the feelings?

The good doesn't remain forever and the challenges don't remain forever.

They are all coming and going.

Life becomes sweeter as you appreciate all of the changes and differences with ease.

IN THE PRESENCE OF WHAT IS

Time: About 7-10 minutes up to as long as you'd like.

If you wanted to shorten this to use at the end of a yoga class, for example, you can trim the pause between questions to thirty seconds to one minute.

Teacher's Note:
This meditation helps guide people back to an enhanced state of being-ness.

Instead of thinking about the past or worrying about the future, this helps them enter a state of is-ness, releasing stress and anxiety so that they can experience calm, peaceful presence.

In a world of constant doing, the internal call to enter a state of BEING intensifies.

We must balance doing with being in order to have the most appreciative, fulfilling life. It's like music.

The space between the musical notes is just as important as the notes themselves.

Start to settle into the natural rise and fall of your breath.

Without going into your past or future, ask yourself what is present for you right now.

Check out whatever you're experiencing in this moment. Welcome whatever you find there.

Is it a thought, a feeling, a sensation? All three?

(Wait about 30 seconds to a minute)

Welcome all of them. Let whatever arises, arise.

Be present with whatever appears, without screening anything out.

Without judgment.

(Wait a minute or two)

Perhaps something is deeper than that.

Ask yourself, "Is there anything underneath the thought, feeling, or sensation? What is deeper than that?"

See what message you receive...

(Wait a minute or two)

Now ask, "Beneath that, what is here that is already complete and whole within me now?"

(Wait a minute or two)

You might notice that your body relaxes, or you tune into your heart more.

You are in a deeper state of BEING-NESS.

You are more awake, aware, and open.

Allow yourself to reside in this state of being-ness for the next ____ *(however long you have allotted for meditation today)*.

GUIDING THEM OUT

As you re-enter your daily experiences, see if you can remain more present with what is.

Instead of judging yourself or others, or thinking about what you or they "should be" feeling or doing,

let go of trying to arrange your experience so that it measures up to some predetermined idea.

This only creates internal struggle.

Instead, welcome the entire range of whatever you're experiencing, moment to moment.

Now you are being in the presence of what is, more relaxed as you experience the ups and downs of life.

SENSES MEDITATION

Time: 8 minutes minimum, up to an hour

Teacher's Note:
You may choose to focus on just one of the senses for the entire
meditation, or explore each of them within the same meditation.

This meditation brings you instantly into your body, grounding you in the
present moment, reducing stress and fear instantly, replacing them with
a deep sense of calm and connection. It is a practice of awareness in its
truest form.

Today we're going to take a journey into each of our senses,

 immersing ourselves in the awareness of what our bodies are
perceiving,

grounding ourselves in the present moment.

This practice is best done seated with an erect spine to tell your
system that you are alert and attentive.

You may choose to put a bolster, pillow, or folded-up blanket
underneath you for support.

If you're experiencing any strain or discomfort, feel free to lie down
on your back instead, placing a bolster or pillow underneath your
knees for support.

Let's begin.

Sense of Smell

Close your eyes and bring your awareness to your nose. Notice what you smell. You might smell laundry detergent on your clothes, lotion on your skin, or deodorant. You might smell the general scent of the room. Stay connected and see if you can notice subtler and subtler scents. If your mind wanders, as soon as you recognize it, bring it back to the sense of smell.

Wait at least 15 seconds, or as long as you like for a longer meditation.

Sense of Taste

Keep your eyes closed and shift your awareness to your tongue. What do you taste? Perhaps something you drank earlier, like coffee or tea, or something you ate. Maybe you brushed your teeth not too long ago, and you can still taste a bit of toothpaste, or you had a mint or piece of gum earlier. As you smell the air around you, this may also provide a subtle taste on your tongue. Continue to focus on your sense of taste.

Wait at least 15 seconds, or as long as you like for a longer meditation.

Sense of Touch

Eyes still closed, notice the places where your body is touching whatever you're sitting or lying on. Without moving, notice what sensations your hands pick up. Feel the clothing on your skin. Feel the subtle weight of any jewelry or accessories that you're wearing. Feel the hair on your head. The hair on your body. Notice what the air feels like on your skin. Focus on the sense of touch.

Wait at least 15 seconds, or as long as you like for a longer meditation.

Sense of Sight

Slowly open your eyes and shift to your sense of sight. Without moving your face, look in any direction that you like and notice what you see. The colors, textures, and shapes of various objects and things around you, your own body. Notice more with your peripheral vision. What other colors or shapes or objects are in your field of awareness? Allow your gaze to soften and go a little hazy for a bit. Gaze more intently now - hyper-focus. Find more intricate patterns and tinier details. Continue to focus on your sense of sight. If your mind wanders, guide it back to noticing what you see.

Wait at least 15 seconds, or as long as you like for a longer meditation.

Sense of Sound *(Modify this to match the sounds in your space. These are suggestions and will differ whether inside or outside).*

Close your eyes and bring your attention to your ears and the sense of sound. What do you hear? If inside: notice the sound of my voice, the music (if using), the air conditioner or fan, the sound of your own breath, or the sound of the breath of the person next to you *(if there is one)*. See if you can hear specific instruments within the music and more minute details.

If outside: notice the sound of the breeze against your ears, the wind through the trees, the birds *(or crickets - if it's evening/night)* chirping, the traffic on the street, or other people walking by. If near water, the sound of the ocean or water fountain. What subtler and subtler textures of sound can you pick out? Stay connected to the sense of sound.

Wait at least 15 seconds, or as long as you like for a longer meditation.

Wipe the slate clean now,
and come back to neutral.

If you chose to utilize more than one,
or all of the senses in your meditation:

Think back. Were any of the senses easier for you to
stay connected to?

GUIDING THEM OUT

This week, as you move through various activities,
see how much you can tune into your senses.

(Or if you selected only one sense for this meditation)
See how much you can continue to tune into the sense of
____ and remain in a state of present awareness.

Take several pauses throughout the day and
simply notice what you're experiencing.

Take some deep breaths and you may find yourself
feeling more relaxed, grounded, and present.

HAMSA MEDITATION

Time: This is a 10-minute meditation that can be shortened or lengthened as desired

---

Teacher's Note:
This meditation helps us remember the deepest truth of who we truly are and revives our connection with universal intelligence.

The Script
So many of us feel disconnected from ALL THAT IS, and unworthy.

Unworthy of love, and unworthy of all the best that life has to offer.

Most often this is due to hurtful experiences from our childhood that causes us to forget our innate awesomeness.

The Hamsa meditation and breathing practice will oxygenate and enliven your body, increase your mental focus, and remind you of your intrinsic worthiness.

The meaning of Hamsa is "I am that."

Just as we are made up of the universe, the universe is within us.

The subatomic particles that make us up, also make up animals, rocks, trees, oceans, the atmosphere, and planets.

The tiniest particles of matter are energy.

We are pure energy, connected to and part of all of the energy within the universe.

Begin with a few deep breaths.

Start to slow down and deepen your breathing.

When you inhale, expand your belly, and

when you exhale, allow your belly to fall.

Continue this pattern for a couple of minutes.

You can close your eyes if you like, or gaze softly downward.

Now, as you inhale, silently, within your mind, think "HAM" (*pronounced hum*).

Pause and hold your breath for a moment, then exhale and think "SA" (*rhymes with ahhh*).

Inhale, expand your stomach, and mentally say HAM.

Exhale, feel your stomach soften, and say to yourself SA.

Repeat for a couple more minutes.

Next, bring your awareness to the base of your spine.

Inhale with the mental sound HAM, and guide your in-breath from the base of your spine up to the crown of your head.

Exhale, with the mental sound SA, guides your out-breath from the crown of your head back down to the base of your spine.

Continue for a couple of minutes.

Lastly, shift your attention to your nostrils.

Inhale, "hear" the mental sound HAM as your breath enters your nose,

Exhale, guide the mental sound SA as you feel the air exiting your nostrils. Continue for two more minutes.

(Sprinkle these in over the next 1-2 minutes)

I am worthy.

I am whole.

I am complete.

I am part of the energy of ALL THAT IS.

Pause for 30 seconds to a minute.

GUIDING THEM OUT

Bring your hands to prayer position.

Guide your thumbs to the center of your eyebrows, the seat of your inner knowing.

Thumbs to the center of your chest, feeling your subtle heartbeat there.

Bow in, chin to chest, and remember that you are made of the same energy that creates worlds.

"I am that."

SA TA NA MA + MUDRA MEDITATION

Time: 10 minutes

Teacher's Note:
This is a great meditation for those who find it challenging to sit still and clear their minds.

It utilizes hand positions that anchor practitioners to Bija mantras (a one-syllable sound used in yoga or meditation practice), deepening their connection to the meaning behind the sounds.

Within a group setting, I have practitioners chant it silently in their minds, as they may go at different speeds.

Alternatively, you could have them chant the bija mantras out loud for added power through the resonance of the sounds.

The Script

The Sa Ta Na Ma Meditation is in Sanskrit, a classical language of India, and utilizes Mudras (hand positions) to invoke meaning.

Not only does this meditation increase mental focus and concentration, but it reminds us of the infinite cycle of life and to recognize discomfort as a signifier of growth.

It consists of one-syllable sounds that we repeat on a loop along with the mudras.

Sa = Infinity. We are energetic beings with consciousness that extends beyond the physical. Energy can never be destroyed.

Ta = Life. Experiencing the whole tapestry of life - happy, sad, good, bad, and everything in between.

Na = Transformation. Period of growth.

Ma = Rebirth. Emerging with new knowledge.

Before we practice the mudras with the mantras and begin our meditation, allow me to share with you The Story of the Lobster:

Lobsters can live up to 100 years old. During the first seven years of life, they molt (shed their old shell) up to 25 times, and once per year after that. As they grow, their shell becomes so tight that further growth is impossible, so they find a safe spot to hide, shed their old shell, and form a new one.

Humans go through this too!

You're going along your life doing just fine when something happens that causes you to halt.

It may be some sort of trauma, a new life stage, or a feeling.

You'll know you're ready for a big growth period because you feel uncomfortable, stuck, and out-of-sorts.

If you recognize this stage for what it is - a springboard to greater understanding and new expansion, it becomes much easier to accept and move through gracefully.

The discomfort signifies that you are ready for a new adventure, job, relationship, interest, or internal shift. This meditation is the perfect reminder of the infinite process of life.

Let's begin by lengthening our spines and taking a few deep breaths.

(Guide three deep breaths)

Press your thumbs against your forefingers and in your mind, say "Sa".

Press your thumbs to your middle fingers and say "Ta".

Press your thumbs to your ring fingers and say "Na".

Press your thumbs to your pinkie fingers and say "Ma".

Remembering their meaning,

press your thumbs to forefingers, "Infinity".

Thumbs to your middle fingers "Life".

Thumbs to your ring fingers, "Transformation".

Thumbs to your pinkie fingers "Rebirth".

Sa...		Sa...		Sa...
Ta...	*Pause* →	Ta...	*Pause* →	Ta...
Na...		Na...		Na...
Ma...		Ma...		Ma...

Continue this pattern for the next ___minutes
(the duration of your meditation. You may also choose to do the mudras for a few minutes, then stop them and continue to meditate in silence).

GUIDING THEM OUT

(If you haven't already, invite students to stop the mudras and mantras now.)

Take some slow, deep breaths into your abdomen, sitting up nice and tall.

Remember the story of the lobster next time you're feeling uncomfortable, out of sorts, or too tight for your shell.

The discomfort may be signifying that you are ready for a new adventure, job, relationship, skill, internal shift, or other change in your life.

Accept the growth stage as a necessary part of your next level of expansion.

SURRENDERING

Time: 10 minutes

Teacher's Note:
This is a great meditation to calm the nervous system and stop trying to control the uncontrollable, allowing our internal security system to sift out of high-alert mode.

By relaxing into the is-ness of the moment, we release our tight grip on things, and sometimes solutions appear organically from this new place.

The Script
Surrendering to relaxation is a practice just like anything else!

Surrendering while breathing can help you let go and feel like you don't have to be on high alert or control everything.

You can experience a physical, mental, emotional, or even spiritual release just by letting go.

This practice is best done while lying down.

Gently make your way onto your back, and feel free to put a bolster or pillow under your knees for support, and maybe even a blanket over you for extra comfort.

Close your eyes.

See if you can expand and lengthen a bit in all directions.

Guide your forehead and chin parallel to the earth.

Allow your feet to fall open. Arms relaxed in a low "V" by your sides, palms facing up.

Relax your body 20% more, and feel the earth supporting you.

Take a slow, deep, full breath in, and let it out with an audible sigh, making an "Ahhhhhhh" sound.

Again, take a slow, deep breath in, and exhale through your mouth, "Ahhhhhhh."

Close your eyes, and turn your vision inward.

Watch your breath and see where it goes.

Follow the oxygen, as if it were visible, as it flows through your body.

Let's assign it a color, a light neon blue. Let's watch the breath as it moves into your lungs.

Breathe in for 4, 3, 2, 1.

And keeping your lips sealed this time, exhale through your nose for 4, 3, 2, 1.

Breathe in for 4, 3, 2, 1.

Breathe out your nose for 4, 3, 2, 1.

Continuing to see the neon light, a little bit slower now...

Breathe in for 5, 4, 3, 2, 1.

Breathe out for 5, 4, 3, 2, 1.

Breathe in for 6, 5, 4, 3, 2, 1.

Breathe out for 6, 5, 4, 3, 2, 1.

Now release the visualization, but continue with these nice long relaxing breaths and just BE HERE.

Feel the gift of your breath. Feel your body settling deeper toward the earth.

Surrender to gravity.

Let go and release a little deeper.

Let go of everything from the past week.

Everything that you don't need anymore.

Anything weighing you down.

Any unpleasant experience you had, not completing everything you wanted to get done, let it go now.

Ask yourself if there is anything you need to forgive someone else or yourself for, and If so, you may think to yourself, "I forgive and release you, as you forgive and release me."

Feel the weight leave your body.

Feel how much more open your body feels now, allowing you to relax even more.

Letting go, letting be.

Letting go, letting be.

Letting go.......I am free.....

Allow yourself to rest, feeling the support of the earth beneath you. The support of the universe within and around you.

Stay here for the next ___ minutes *(however long you have allotted for this meditation today).*

GUIDING THEM OUT

Take a slow, deep, full breath in, and let it out with an audible sigh, making an "Ahhhhhhh" sound.

Again, take a slow, deep breath in, and exhale through your mouth, "Ahhhhhhh."

As you bring your awareness back, consider what else in your life you would like to surrender to.

Is there something that you've felt constricted around, trying to make happen, but you feel like you're just hitting your head against the wall?

Once you surrender to the is-ness of it, a new question appears.

From this new place, Is there anything that feels like right action now?

You may not get an answer right away, but sometimes it will appear within the next couple of weeks, often while you're doing some mundane task.

OCEAN OF ENERGY

Time: 10 min

Teacher's note:

This one is best done while lying down on the back. If you have access to props, use them as listed below.

This meditation invites practitioners to explore quantum physics at its best: helping us remember that we are immersed within, and an integral part of the fundamental energy that makes up the universe.

The Script

For this meditation, lie down on your back with your feet a bit wider than your hips.

You may enjoy a bolster or pillow underneath your knees, a blanket over your body, and a hand towel or eye mask covering your eyes.

Lengthen your entire body, creating a bit more space in your spine.

Allow your toes to relax outwards.

Arms down by your sides, palms facing up. Close your eyes.

Take a few deep breaths.

Inhale, allow your belly and chest to rise; exhale, and allow your belly to soften.

Inhale, slow and deep, exhale long and complete.

Once more, inhale, expand, and exhale soften.

Imagine that your body is a sponge.

Weightless...

On a sea of prana, a sea of pure energy...

Have you ever experienced a day at the pool or ocean where the sunlight glimmers through the water? See the energy sparkle.

Feel the slight rocking motion of the sea beneath you.

You begin to soak in the sea, drifting down. Becoming immersed. Filling up with energy.

Feeling totally held, nurtured, and completely at peace.

Pretty soon you are completely submerged.

You can feel the gentle rocking motion of the sea within you.

Pure energy.

You are the sea. The sea is you.

You are the energy remembering itself.

Drifting. Timeless.

Pure Energy.

Remain for the next ___ minutes.
(as long as you have allotted for this meditation)

GUIDING THEM OUT

When you're ready to return, gently guide your awareness back to your body.

Feel the floor beneath you.

The gravity that allows you to sense yourself again.

Gently roll to one side, and press your top hand into the floor to help you rise to a seated position.

Slowly allow your eyes to take on light.

Allow this meditation to serve as a reminder that you are connected to and made of the same energy that creates worlds.

You are a singular expression of the infinite. Because of this, you are always enough, and you inherently belong.

ENERGY HEALING

Time: 10 minutes, but can allow more time for resting in silence afterward.

Teacher's Note:

The most recent data shows that the placebo effect cure rate is between 15% and 72%.

The power of the body-mind connection through intention, meditation, prayer, and belief is miraculous! This meditation will assist practitioners to engage their own healing power.

The Script

Lengthen your spine, draw your shoulder blades down a bit to open your chest, and face your palms up.

Close your eyes. Become aware of your breath.

Guide a deeper inhale into your lungs, using your diaphragm, exhale let it go nice and easy.

With every inhale Imagine bringing vital energy into your system.

With every exhale imagine releasing any accumulated toxins and stress.

Inhale, fill up your belly then chest to full capacity.

Exhale, and release every last bit of your breath slowly and completely.

Stay with this breath for the next ten deep inhales and exhales.

(Guide the sound of the breath, counting down)

10

9

8

7

6

5

4

3

2

1

Now keep breathing into your belly but allow your subconscious mind to take over your breath.

Imagine a bright white light glowing above your head.

Draw this light through the crown of your head.

Allow it to extend into your face, neck, shoulders, arms, torso, hips, and legs.

Extending all the way through your fingers and toes.

Your entire body is now lit up with bright healing light that extends about five inches around your entire being.

Every cell in your system is now vibrating with this energy.

If there is part of you that needs healing, whether an old or recent injury, an illness or disease, a broken heart, a negative thought pattern that runs your mind, migraines, etc., guide your awareness to the part of you that is most connected to the symptoms you are experiencing.

Imagine the light growing even brighter there, warming, heating the area.

If you understand the specifics of the injury, illness, or disease that you're experiencing, imagine the healing process taking place within your cells, step by step.

You may even hear or imagine a sound, a tone, as this energy heals the area.

You could say to your highest self, "If this healing has a sound, allow me to hear the sound now."

Even if there is not something specific to heal at this time, then just bask in this healing light that is purifying, energizing, and brings your cells to full vibrancy.

Receive this upgrade.

Once this process feels complete, say to yourself, "I am now healed and energized, and I am so grateful and thankful for this healing."

Remain basking in white light a bit longer.

You may notice a feeling of vibrant, buzzing, alive energy, or a sense of deep relaxation, or bliss.

(Wait about a minute)

GUIDING THEM OUT

Begin to tune into your breathing again.

Deep inhale into your belly, then chest.

Exhaling, releasing air from your chest and then your belly.

Guide your hands to your heart in prayer position.

Bow in, chin to chest, in gratitude for the harmony you now experience throughout your entire being.

RAINBOW COLOR MEDITATION

Time: 10 minutes with the option to stay longer

Teacher's Note:
This magical meditation utilizes breath, visualization, and calling in sensation, allowing one to embody the qualities of each rainbow color and culminates in a grand finale of awesomeness.

The Script:

Close your eyes, lengthen your spine, and take a slow, deep breath in through your nose, and exhale, letting go. Take a deep breath in, from the bottom to the top of your lungs, and let it go. Deep breath in, belly, chest, and let it go.

On your next breath, breathe in the color red, and then continue to breathe naturally. Imagine the color infusing your body, permeating every cell, bringing with it a sense of inner strength and stability. Safety and security. For a few moments, stay with the color red.

Wait for about 30 seconds to allow time to experience.

Breathe out the color red, and breathe in bright, vibrant orange. Allow orange to encapsulate your body, providing a sense of warmth, comfort, and utter well-being. Continue breathing, visualizing, and feeling the orange color.

Wait for about 30 seconds to allow time to experience.

Breathe out the color orange, and breathe in the color yellow. Bright and radiant, bonding with your entire being a sense of happiness, confidence, and a deeper connection to your unique signature of creative power. Reside within the color yellow as you breathe.

Wait for about 30 seconds to allow time to experience.

Breathe out the color yellow, and breathe in the color green.
Beautiful emerald green that brings with it a sense of regeneration and renewed health. Repairing and revitalizing your cells, bringing your system back to balance. Remain with the color green as you breathe.

Wait for about 30 seconds to allow time to experience.

Breathe out the color green, and breathe in the color blue. A deep blue encapsulates your body, providing a sense of calmness and peace. Feel this cool inner peace as you breathe.

Wait for about 30 seconds to allow time to experience.

Breathe out the color blue, and breathe in the color purple. Purple permeates your system and you feel this color providing a greater connection to your intuition and higher consciousness. Clearing out anything clouding your clarity of purpose. Stay with the color purple as you reconnect to your deeper sense of inner knowing.

Wait for about 30 seconds to allow time to experience.

Breathe out the color purple, and breathe in the color of iridescent white. White coats your body and fills every cell. This luminous color connects you to the grid of energy of all that is. You feel your connection strengthen, which allows you to vibrate at the highest frequency available to you now. Energized and connected to unlimited energy. Stay with the color white as you breathe.

Wait for about 30 seconds to allow time to experience.

Breathe out the color white and now take in the full rainbow spectrum. The beautiful, magical, awe-inspiring mystery of life that encompasses you and everything around you. Take it in. Feel it infuse you and enliven you. Remain here for a few more minutes, resting in this magic.

Wait for a minute or two (or add time here if you want to have a longer meditation).

GUIDING THEM OUT

Bring your awareness back to your breath, and slowly open your eyes.

Notice this fully balanced and optimized state that you have created through the power of your breath, visualization, and the embodiment of specific qualities and sensations.

Take this with you throughout your day (or into dreamland if you are headed to sleep soon).

HEART OPENING

Time: about 10 minutes with the option to allow more time to rest in silence afterward.

Teacher's Note:

This is a great meditation to offer on or around Valentine's Day, or if you're a yoga teacher, in conjunction with a class focus on heart openers/ backbends.

The Script:

Close your eyes and bring your awareness to your breath.

Expand your belly using your diaphragm when you inhale, and soften your belly down towards the earth at the end of your exhale. Let your inhale expand from the bottom of your lungs all the way to the top, lifting and expanding your chest, then softening back down as you exhale. Inhale belly, chest. Exhale letting go, letting go, letting go. Allow your breath to shift to automatic now.

Let your awareness settle in your heart. Notice if it feels tight or expansive, light or heavy. Be open to any thoughts or sensations that arise. Keep the awareness around your heart space, and notice what you find there.

Ask if your heart has something to tell you; a message that you need to receive. Be open to different kinds of messages. It may be a word or a phrase, a symbol, a color, or a sound. Just open up to receive for the next 30 seconds.

(Wait 30 seconds)

If your heart feels light, expansive, warm, and open, you may wish to reside right here for the remainder of this meditation. Continue to sense these sensations, deepening your ability to give and receive love freely. You may choose to send love to someone who needs it, or even to a group of people.

If your heart feels heavy, closed off, or you feel nothing at all, then consider that we often build a protective wall around our hearts after we've been hurt. You may choose to visualize it in your mind's eye as a wall around your heart, made of bricks that were placed there little by little throughout your life as you experienced emotionally painful things.

Though this wall protects you from feeling the intensity of uncomfortable emotions, this wall also closes you off from joy and higher love. Know now, that you are much stronger than you were before. You have had so many experiences. You have gained knowledge, and have more tools. You have much more inner strength and resilience than you did before.

Perhaps you are willing to let some old hurts and resentments go now. Maybe you're willing to release this cumbersome burden you've been carrying around. Consider that in order to experience great love, there is a risk involved because we can't control other people, and sometimes love fades or changes. But even so, you are brave enough to handle whatever comes your way, and it is worth the risk to experience deep love rather than hardening your heart and shutting down for the rest of your life.

You may choose to visualize removing some, many, or even all of the bricks from around your heart one by one. Take a few moments to do this now.

(Wait 15 seconds)

After the bricks are removed, sense or imagine that your heart feels lighter, freer, and open. The area around your heart feels peaceful and warm and relaxed.

This new openness feels really good, really expansive. Chest soft, heart soft. Warm and bright. Your whole being feels light and free.

Allow yourself to explore these feelings and sensations for a bit...

(Wait the desired amount of time)

Now it's time for a choice:

You can choose to stay with your heart open and expansive...

or you can protect yourself again by replacing some or all of the bricks around your heart again...

Or maybe a third option...

You replace it with thinner, lighter bricks now, or some other material altogether, like silk or crystal.

Know that you can come back to this meditation whenever you like and make a new choice.

See that the choice is always there.

GUIDING THEM OUT

Begin to take some deeper breaths.

Draw your awareness back to the present moment.

Allow yourself a few more moments of stillness.

Notice how you feel, if you sense any difference within your being after this experience.

Open your eyes as you bring your hands to your chest in prayer position.

Bow in, chin to chest, honoring your magnificent heart.

CALLING IN LOVE

Time: 10 min

> *Teacher's Note:*
> *Here's another great meditation for Valentine's Day, Couples Retreats or workshops, or if a yoga teacher, in conjunction with a class themed around heart openers/backbends.*

The Script:

Close your eyes and focus on your breath going in and out. Allow your breath to come and go with less effort and more flow. Relax, and watch your breath.

Now allow yourself to become more still. Feel yourself settling into a deeper sense of calmness.

Bring your awareness to your heart. Imagine that you feel a sensation of warmth within and around the area of your heart.

Ask yourself this question. You may hear it as words, or see the words written across your field of your consciousness.

"WHAT IS ESSENTIAL TO ME IN A LOVING RELATIONSHIP?"

For example, things like: Humor, kindness, fun, tenderness, chemistry, and similar views.... Allow your own words to appear.

Your mind may distract you. That's okay. If you notice you've drifted from the question, gently nudge yourself back to consider what you find most important.

Are these qualities that others have said you should want, or does this accurately represent what you really want, in your deepest heart?

Reassess.

Confirm.

If you are in a relationship now, ask yourself if these are things that are present between you. Are you honoring your deepest heart?

Now shift to you.

Know that receiving love from someone else will never fill the void of YOU NOT LOVING YOU. Are you honoring yourself with the same qualities you want in a relationship with someone else?

Are you being kind to yourself?

Are you showing up for yourself?

Are you being loving with yourself?

Do you trust yourself?

Are you being honest with yourself?

Are you having fun?

Notice your answers to these questions. How you treat yourself sets the bar for what you allow from others. Talk to yourself as you would someone you deeply love. Be true to yourself. Know yourself intimately. Trust yourself. Accept and love yourself without conditions.

Breathe in, and breathe out. Relax. Silently say to yourself, "No matter what happened in the past, or what I did or didn't do, I deeply love, appreciate, and accept myself. I am now ready, willing, and able to co-create a loving relationship."

GUIDING THEM OUT

Take a few more deep breaths.

Place your hands at your heart, and bow in honor of the messages you received from your heart during this meditation today, the love you are calling into your life, and the love that exists within you.

SENDING LOVE

Time: 10 minutes

Teacher's Note:

This meditation provides the medium to connect us more deeply to our hearts and to others by sending love to those we feel closest to, those who live in a place in the world that needs some extra healing right now, someone we're having difficulty with, and to all beings everywhere, including ourselves. When we focus on the love we have for others, we experience a greater sense of ease, comfort, and good feelings, and general stress often disappears.

This meditation is best done while seated.

The Script:

Begin this meditation by closing your eyes, lifting your breastbone, and lengthening your spine, inviting in a sense greater spaciousness.

For the next minute or two, simply focus on your breath coming in, and your breath going out.

Without trying to control your breath in any way, just observe it.

Allow yourself to lose sense of time and distractions.

(Wait 2 minutes)

Bring your palms to your chest in prayer position and place your thumbs in the groove of your breastbone. Begin to sense your heartbeat.

Now rub your palms together to generate sensation and heat.

When they are very warm, place one palm, and then the other, over your heart.

Guide warm energy from your heart through your arms to your hands back into your heart.

Heart, arms, hands, heart.

Continue this looped circuit of energy for a minute.

(Wait 1 minute)

Send this warmth throughout your entire body now.

Allow the feeling to spread like warm honey throughout your system.

Your whole being fills up with this loving heart energy, providing a sense of contentment, bliss, ...maybe even euphoria.

Next, cup your hands underneath your heart.

Visualize heart energy flowing from your palms outward to those you feel closest to, which may include your current family, family of origin, friends, and other loved ones.

Now send love outward to someone you are having difficulty with.

If there's no one you're currently having difficulty with, send it to someone you had difficulty with from your past.

Even if they have passed away, you can still send them love.

Imagine an image of them out in front of you and send a warm beam of love.

Send love to those in a part of the world that needs extra support right now.

Then send loving energy out into the universe, to all beings everywhere.

Lastly, it's time to receive.

It's a flow of energy, like an infinity loop: I give, I receive, I give, I receive, I give, I receive.

Allow a wave of energy to flow back to your heart.

Receive the love as it comes back to you.

Place one palm, then the other, over your heart, in gratitude, feeling the warmth generated there.

GUIDING THEM OUT

Bring your hands to prayer position at your chest, placing your thumb knuckles at the groove of your breastbone.

Notice how you feel after completing this meditation.

When you're in the vibration of love, you are connected to who you truly are.

And it is through this highest vibration, that you are always connected to your innermost self, your loved ones, and all beings everywhere.

INNER BODY SENSING

Time: 5-10 min

Teacher's Note:

This meditation is really good for helping people experience and connect to their bodies by tuning into the subtle energy within. It brings a greater sense of present awareness and focus, and feels pretty magical ;)

The Script:

Lengthen your spine and turn your palms to face upward.

Begin to breathe deeply and fully.

Bring your awareness to your chest.

Feel the subtle feeling of energy there.

Not in your mind, but go right to the place itself. Feel the vibration and sensation of energy. It may feel slightly tingly.

Let's broaden the sensation.

From there, radiate the energy outwards in all directions. Throughout your torso. Send the sensation down your legs, from your chest through your arms, and up into your throat all the way to your head.

Can you sense the aliveness?

The tingly sensation, the subtle vibration of energy that exists within you? This total body sensation flowing through you is Prana, Qi, Lifeforce.

Reside in this sensation, experiencing the vibrant energy of life that flows through you for the next ___minutes *(as long as you've allotted for meditation)*.

GUIDING THEM OUT

Guide your awareness to your lungs.

Take some slow, deep breaths into the lower portion of your lungs and fill all the way up to your chest.

Reach your arms over your head and stretch, squeezing your muscles.

Open your eyes.

As you move through your week getting caught up with all the DOING, intermittently take a minute to tune in and feel the energy within your body.

This guides you into a state of present awareness, a state of BEING.

By remaining present within yourself, you may even notice that you are connecting more deeply with others and, in general, connecting more deeply with life.

LONG MEDITATIONS
(10-35 minutes)

These meditations are 10 - 35 minutes. By inviting more time for quiet near the end, they can go even longer if you like.

BODY SCAN FOR RELAXATION

Time: 10-20 minutes

Teacher's Note:

Just as there are visual, auditory, and kinesthetic learners, the same goes for meditators.

Some may find it easier to focus on words or music, some on visualizations, and others on sensations within their bodies.

This meditation provides a kinesthetic exploration of each body part, allowing them to release any tension that they find along the way.

In addition, it's really helpful for those who have a very busy mind and a challenging time sitting for meditation because it gives the mind specific things to do.

This meditation is best done while lying down.

The Script:

If we released built-up tension and stress on a daily basis, imagine how much better we would feel.

By practicing bringing awareness to, and relaxing each part of our bodies, toe to head, we can experience all kinds of releases - mental, emotional, physical, and sometimes even spiritual.

In any case, this practice is sublimely restorative, calms the nervous system, and is great for learning to tune in without judgment.

For this meditation lie down on your back. Feel free to put a bolster or pillow underneath your knees for added comfort.

If you would like to get extra cozy, you can drape a blanket over yourself and cover your eyes with an eye mask.

Close your eyes.

First, notice the places where you feel your body touching the floor. Take a few slow, deep breaths. Inhale through your nose, and exhale through your mouth, making a "haaaaaaa" sound.

Allow yourself to sink a little deeper into the earth. At this moment, know that everything is alright. You have allotted this time to take care of yourself.

There is nowhere else you need to be and nothing else you need to do right now.

As we move through this practice, you might notice that your attention drifts in and out. You may hear my voice, and then it may fade into the background.

All of this is okay. You will hear what you need to hear.

There is nothing you have to do to get this right. You are safe and supported as we enter the space for deep rest and rejuvenation.

As I bring your attention to different parts of your body, allow yourself to feel the sensation there. Notice what's present.

If you notice any pain or tension, just do your best to soften and relax the area.

[Say these words with a very relaxed tone, using a slow pace.]

We'll begin with your right foot. Feel the top of your foot, the sole of your foot, your heel, and your ankle. Feel your shin, your calf, the back of your knee, and your kneecap. Your right thigh and hip, the back of your right thigh/your hamstrings. Bring your awareness to your right buttock.

Release any tension that you find there, and anywhere throughout your right leg and foot.

Now bring your attention to your left foot. Feel the top of your foot, the sole of your foot, your heel, and your ankle. Feel your shin, your calf, the back of your knee, and your kneecap.

Your left thigh and hip, the back of your left thigh/your hamstrings. Bring your awareness to your left buttock. Relax any tension that you find there, and anywhere throughout your left leg and foot.

Feel your pelvis. Relax the lowest part of your belly, your tailbone, and your low back.

Feel your midsection, your stomach.

Release any tension there.

Relax your mid-back.

Feel your heart.

Feel your open chest.

Feel your shoulder blades and your upper back.

Arrive at your shoulders.

If you notice tension there or any other place within your torso, release and let go.

Notice the notch at the base of your throat.

As you bring awareness to your neck, soften the ligaments and tendons.

Allow the back of your head to surrender to gravity a bit more.

Soft cheeks and jaw. Soft mouth. Notice your gums and your teeth.

The inside of your cheeks. Feel your tongue relax in your mouth.

Feel your nose. Your left nostril, your right nostril.

Bring your awareness to your right ear, then your left ear.

Feel both of your ears at the same time.

Relax the skin around your eyes.

Notice your eyelids.

Feel your eyelashes.

Notice your right eye, your left eye.

Allow both eyes to rest in their sockets.

Soften your eyebrows and forehead.

Feel your whole face, your head.

Feel the hairs on your head.

Bring your awareness to the crown of your head. Relaxing everything.

Now imagine pouring your awareness like warm shimmery liquid starting at the crown of your head moving all the way down your entire body to your feet.

Filling up your entire body. **Feel the sensation of your energy throughout your whole being.**

Feel all the parts together now as a whole.

Feeling the entirety of your being.

(You may choose to wait anywhere from 1-5 minutes)

Allow yourself to bask in this sensation for the next ___ minutes.

GUIDING THEM OUT

It's now time to complete this relaxation and awareness practice.

Gently rock your head from side to side.

Take some deeper breaths into your body.

Wriggle your fingers and toes. Stretch your arms above your head, and your toes away from your arms, full morning stretch style.

Yawn if you'd like to take in a little more oxygen. Open your eyes and gently roll to whatever side is calling your name.

Use your top hand to lift yourself up to a seat.

Sit cross-legged, bring your hands to prayer position at your heart, in honor of this time you've set aside to take care of your body and mind in this special way.

PROGRESSIVE MUSCLE RELAXATION

Time: 10 - 20 minutes

Teacher's Note:
This meditation is especially effective for those who find it challenging to sit still.

It gives the mind something to focus on and helps them feel their body.

Many of us hold tension in our bodies on a regular basis. This practice has us squeeze the muscles even more, and then totally let go. By squeezing and then releasing, each part of our bodies feel acknowledged.

In addition, those who tend to disassociate or feel anxious when overly stressed can receive the grounding benefits of this practice so that they can relax and feel safe within their own bodies.

The Script:
This meditation is excellent for releasing accumulated tension and stress held in the body.

We'll be journeying through the body, as I guide you to squeeze and release certain muscles as we go.

To begin, lie down on your back with your feet a bit wider than hip-width apart, arms down by your sides, and palms facing up.

Lengthen your entire body a couple more inches.

Draw the wingtips of your shoulder blades underneath you to help open your chest. Close your eyes.

Bring your attention to your right foot. Point your right toes strongly, curl them under, and squeeze your foot muscles.

Release.

Now flex your ankle, bringing your toes towards your shin bone, engage your calf, and open all of your toes.

Relax.

Squeeze your right kneecap, right thigh, right hamstring, and right buttock.

Release.

Shift your awareness to your left foot. Point your left toes powerfully, curl them under and squeeze the muscles. Now flex your ankle, draw your toes towards your shinbone, and tighten your calf. Fan open all of your toes, even the pinkie toes.

Release.

Engage all the muscles around your left kneecap, squeeze your left thigh, hamstrings, and buttock.

Release.

Make a fist with your right hand, squeeze your fingers together into a tight ball. Engage your forearm, squeeze the muscles around your elbow. Squeeze your biceps, triceps, and right shoulder.

Relax.
Bring your attention to your left hand.

Make a fist and squeeze it tight. Engage your left forearm, elbow, squeeze all of the muscles around your upper arm and left shoulder.

Release.

Squeeze your lower torso including low belly and lower back. Firm all the muscles there.

Release.

Draw in your low ribs, and engage your mid-abdominals and mid-back. Circumferentially draw in your waistline.

Release.

Squeeze your chest and upper back muscles. Hug the muscles around your heart from the front, sides, and back.

Release.

Gently tighten your neck muscles.

Relax.

Squeeze your face. Bring your features to the middle of your face and scrunch it up like you are tasting a super-sour lemon. Now open your mouth wide, stretch your jaw, open your eyes wide, and squeeze the muscles around your ears and your entire head.

Release.

Now squeeze your entire body. Tighten your core, squeeze your stomach muscles, squeeze your chest, press your shoulder blades down, straighten your arms, make fists, squeeze your buttocks, and your thighs, flex your ankles, and open your toes.

Release.

Now check to see if there is any residual tension left anywhere in your body.

If you find a place where there is still tension, ask it if it has a message for you, then wait...and listen...and receive what's there.

Squeeze all of the muscles around it to signify that it's been heard.

Release the muscle engagement.

Take a deep, full belly inhale, then audibly exhale through your mouth, making a "haaaaa" sound.

Another deep inhale, exhale open mouth, let it go.

Allow your entire body to go completely slack.

Soften everything, surrender to gravity.

And finally, relax your mental muscles. Feel the spaciousness you've created both in your body and your mind.

Allow yourself to rest in stillness for the next ___ minutes
(the remaining time you've allotted for meditation).

GUIDING THEM OUT

Start to bring your awareness back.

Stretch your arms above your head, and yawn, taking in more oxygen.

Roll onto one side, in fetal position.

Open your eyes, and press your top hand into the earth to help yourself up to a seated posture.

Bring your hands to your heart, in gratitude for all that your body does for you each day, and for your ability to generate this state of inner ease and relaxation.

HEALING HANDS MEDITATION

Time: 10 - 15 minutes

Teacher's Note:

This meditation often surprises people in the best way because they FEEL the energy within their hands and can sense and play with an actual ball of energy.

For some, it's the first eye-opening, mind-expanding experience that helps them truly understand that we are energetic beings.

The look of wonder on students' faces as they explore this practice is so cool to witness, and I love the responses I hear from students afterward.

The Script:

Everything in the universe is made up of energy, and we are too.

At the subatomic level, a wave becomes a particle when it's observed. The observer creates reality. This coupled with the fact that placebos heal people demonstrates that we have within us the power to heal ourselves.

This meditation allows you to slow down, explore the sensation of energy, and utilize the power of your focused intention to guide the energy to a place within you that needs healing.

This creates a field of potential in which healing can occur. You might be amazed that you can actually feel the energy between your hands if you have never done something like this before!

Begin seated in any position that is comfortable for you.

You can place a bolster or cushion underneath your hips for added support if you like.

With your arms shoulder-width apart, bend your elbows and fling your wrists vigorously as if you're shaking water off of your hands *(about fifteen times)*.

Now bring your palms together and rub them as you would while trying to keep warm.

Rub them faster, and faster, and faster still.

Feel the warmth you're generating.

Keep rubbing until your hands feel really warm and your arms start to fatigue.

Now go back to the "flinging off water" motion about fifteen times, then rub your hands together in order to stimulate heat and sensation in your hands again.

Keep going, keep going, faster, faster, faster.

Next, bring your hands out in front of you, about twelve inches apart, palms facing one another.

Close your eyes and keep them closed for the remainder of this meditation.

Moving very slowly, almost imperceptibly, guide your hands to about two inches apart.

Stay there for a few moments.

Then very, very slowly, like in a slow-motion video, draw your hands back to about 12 inches apart.

You may notice a sensation like pulling taffy or a slight magnetic pull.

In super slow motion, draw your hands back to about two inches apart.

It may feel almost as if there is something in between your hands. Like the air feels "firmer" somehow.

Do this a few more times.

Now bring your hands about six or seven inches apart.

Imagine you're holding a ball of energy.

Slowly guide one hand over the ball and one hand underneath it.

You can choose to add color if you like.

It might be a glowing white or golden light, or blue, green, yellow, violet....any color that comes to mind.

Gradually guide your hands to the sides of this energy ball now.

Feel around its shape. Notice what it feels like to you, its qualities.

Wherever your hands are, pause, and bring to mind something within you that requires healing.

It may be an old or recent injury, an illness, or disease, a broken heart, headaches/migraines, a poor digestive system, negative thoughts, or anything else.

Guide your awareness to the place where you experience symptoms the most.

Gently move your hands to the nearest position that you can get to this area.

Place your hands on this spot. Imagine with as many details as you can, as clearly as you can, using all of your senses, a healing taking place.

For example, If you have a torn ligament in your knee, imagine the ligament re-knitting together. The fibers reattaching stronger than ever. As your hands continue to send healing energy to the area, you may notice that it feels a bit tingly, cool, or even warm.

See in your mind's eye, the healing occurring.

Imagine going to the doctor or physical therapist and how they are shocked by this healing, the new range of motion you have, and new things that you can do.

Imagine testing your knee out - bending it back and forth and doing various activities. Get into the feeling of it.

How you feel when your knee feels great and you can do all the things you want to do.

Take about a minute to visualize as many rich details as you can.

(Wait one minute)

GUIDING THEM OUT

Honor the amazing capacity within you to heal by slowly bringing your hands to prayer position at your breastbone, in gratitude for this healing.

When you're ready, open your eyes.

MOUNTAIN MEDITATION

Time: 15 minutes. Can allow more time at the end to rest in silence.

Teacher's Note:

In a world filled with judgments, this meditation helps us realize that the opinions of others have nothing to do with us.

At our core, we are already whole and complete.

We are awesome, magnificent, and awe-inspiring through all seasons of our lives, no matter what is going on around us.

The Script:

Lengthen your spine, close your eyes, and guide some slow, even breaths into your body.

Begin to form an image in your mind of the most magnificent, beautiful mountain that you can imagine.

This mountain will be experiencing all kinds of weather, including snow, so keep that in mind as you bring this image to life.

It might be a place you've visited or a mountain that you've seen in an image or a movie. Let it come into focus; add in more subtle details.

Start to sense its overall shape - its wide base rooted in the earth's crust, soft rolling hills, or steep peaks that extend high into the sky.

Feel how massive it is.

How solid, unmoving, and beautiful. Feel these mountain-like qualities within your own body.

As if you and the mountain are becoming one.

Share its massiveness and stillness.

Within this stillness become the mountain.

With each breath you take, feel your unwavering stability and timelessness.

Grounded, centered, unmoving. Beyond thoughts and words.

Become aware of the sensation of the traveling sun.

The warm, soft light turns bright and intense, then fades into shadows and finally darkness.

The night sky studded with sparkling stars. There you are, experiencing all of it moment by moment.

The cycle that brings light to dark, dark to light.

In the summer, the sun bakes the dirt and rocks, animals slow down in the heat, and trees and shrubs soak in the sun's rays.

In the fall, some leaves change color. The air is cool and crisp. Animals prepare for winter by storing up.

As winter comes, snow falls, covering the trees and the ground like a soft blanket, and ice forms underneath. Animals hibernate, and quiet sets in.

Spring brings new life, melting ice that turns into waterfalls, and wildflowers pop up. Birds sing, and insects hum.

The grass, bushes, and trees soak up gentle rain and turn vibrantly green.

The mountain experiences changing weather from moment to moment and month to month.

Its surfaces change and the activities on it change, but it is always being itself.

People come to visit to see the sights and hike the craggy hills.

Some comment on how beautiful it is or what a great day it is to visit.

Others say the trails are too easy or too challenging. That the day is too cold and rainy, or too hot.

None of this matters as at all times the mountain remains its essential self.

The magnificence, magic, and beauty are not changed one bit by whether people see it or not, or what tourists say about it.

It just sits, being itself, unmoved by what happens on the surface.

Allow yourself to remain in this state of steady ongoingness for a few more minutes.

(Wait for 2 minutes)

GUIDING THEM OUT

Begin to bring your awareness back to your body.

Take in some deeper breaths, feeling your belly rise and fall....*(wait for a few moments)*.

If you're lying down, gently turn to one side, open your eyes, and when you feel ready, help yourself up to a seat with a tall spine.

Just like the mountain, we can embody the same central, unwavering stillness and groundedness in the face of everything that changes in our own lives over seconds, hours, and years.

In our lives, and even in our meditation practice, we experience the constantly changing nature of our mind, body, and outer world.

We see that we have our own periods of light and darkness, activity and inactivity, moments of color, and moments of drabness.

We experience storms of varying intensity with our bodies and minds. We endure periods of darkness and pain, as well as elation and joy.

Even our appearance changes constantly.

By embodying the mountain, we connect to our own strength and stability.

We realize that we too can encounter each moment with mindfulness, equanimity, and clarity.

It helps us see that our thoughts, feelings, preoccupations, emotional storms, and the things that happen to us are very much like the weather on the mountain.

We tend to take it all personally, but it is usually impersonal.

The weather of our own lives is not to be ignored or denied, it is to be encountered, honored, felt, known for what it is, and observed as it passes by.

In this way, we come to understand and embody the wisdom that mountains have to teach us.

SPACE TRAVEL

Time: 15 minutes.

Teacher's Note:
When people experience this meditation their problems often become less significant in the face of the vastness of the universe.

They usually feel much lighter, freer, and a bit floaty and dreamy after this one. When meditation is over, invite them to wake up a bit before operating any heavy machinery like a car! ;)

This one is best practiced while lying down. If meditators have access to the following, offer that they put a pillow or bolster underneath their knees, a blanket over their bodies, and cover their eyes with a hand towel or eye mask.

Speak slowly, allowing time in between your words for the experience. If you're guiding this outdoors, remove the verbiage about passing through the roof.

The Script:
Begin this meditation lying down on your back.

Broaden your chest, palms facing up.

Close your eyes.

Take some slow, steady, belly breaths.

Relax your body 20% more.

Use your exhales to release any tension that you find in your body.

As this tension leaves, your body feels lighter as if you feel gravity lessening.

You are becoming lighter still.

You begin to feel weightless.

So weightless that you gently lift off of the ground and begin floating.

You float upwards to the ceiling *(if there is one)*.

Your atomic particles shift through the ceiling and you find that you are now above the roof.

Go a bit higher than that.

Direct your attention downwards and notice what things look like from this perspective.

The buildings, the roads, the cars, bicycles, people, grass, trees, dogs, and birds.

What other things do you notice?

Gently float higher now into the clouds.

Notice the cool, misty quality as you pass through them....heading into the stratosphere.

Higher still into deeper layers of the atmosphere. Amongst the stars now. So beautiful. Twinkling lights everywhere.

Allow yourself to float among them for a while....

(wait for a minute or two)

You may notice our solar system, the milky way.

You may wish to explore some familiar constellations, the planets, or even head towards the sun.

Our solar system is such a small speck within the vastness of the universe.

You may find yourself drawn to other galaxies, planets you've never seen before.

Allow yourself to drift.

Allow yourself to explore.

(wait for a few minutes)

GUIDING THEM OUT

Now it is time to begin heading back.

Start drifting towards our solar system.

Feel yourself drawn towards the earth.

Gently, no rush.

Notice what our beautiful planet looks like from above.

Imagine that this is your first time seeing Earth.

The cloud coverage, then landmasses, the expansive oceans.

As you get closer, you see its greenery, the brown and snow-capped mountains.

Drift slowly towards your country, then your city.

Locate your neighborhood and the place where you started this journey.

Notice the perspective from above.

Head towards the roof. Pass through the roof, and like a feather, wafting towards the spot that you left at the beginning of your journey.

Sense your body weighted with gravity again.

Imagine this is your first breath and guide a slow, long breath into your lungs.

Draw a few more, nice and deep, full and complete. Imagine this is the first time feeling your body.

What does it feel like to be in this body?

Stretch in any way that feels good, and squeeze your muscles if you like.

Take a yawn, letting in more oxygen.

When you're ready, roll to one side.

Wriggle your fingers and toes.

Take your time getting up.

Arrive in a seated position of your choosing.

Lengthen your spine, sitting up nice and tall.

This meditation can leave you with a sense of timelessness or ongoingness, so look all around you and re-orient yourself in this time and space.

Bring your hands to your breastbone in prayer position.

As you go through the next few days, see if you can stay connected to a sense of wonder at the vastness of it all.

Look up at the stars at night.

During the day, what if you looked at a bird or a butterfly as if it was your first time seeing one?

What if you remember how lucky you are to travel around the sun with this family of yours and you tell them that?

What does it feel like to remember that you are made up of the same elements as everything in the vastness of the universe?

What other insights can you take with you from your journey into space?

MY TRUE SELF

Time: about 10-20 minutes

Teacher's Note:

This meditation is for helping people strip down and get naked! Not like that! Haha! But rather stripping away the labels and identifiers that keep people stuck in a box and unavailable for growth.

By getting to the root of their core self, there is a greater connection to the deeper truth of who they really are: one that is ALREADY perfect, whole, complete, lovable, and 100% worthy.

Summarize or read this first part of this script as a precursor to the meditation, then have meditators close their eyes.

When we're babies, we learn our names.

Parents and caregivers help us associate ourselves in relationship to things. "Danny's toy," "Danny's stuffed animal," "Danny's book."

We begin to identify things with ourselves, and we bind them with our sense of who we are.

As we grow, others have opinions and observations about us that they share out loud like, "Wow Danny, you're such a great artist! Or, "Danny, you really need to watch what you're eating, because you're getting fat."

Or "Danny doesn't like to go places because he's so shy."

We add labels to ourselves based on these comments and create more of our own. "I'm a great artist," "I'm fat," "I'm shy," "I'm introverted."

We also have roles that we play: sister/brother, daughter/son, mother/father, grandparent, friend, employer/employee, student, athlete, etc.

We also identify with the activities and jobs that we do: I'm the taxi for my kids, I'm the one who fixes things around the house, I'm the one who keeps everything running, I'm the family connector who plans all the gatherings, etc.

When we hold on to identifiers, we suffer when we lose things.

Who am I if I can no longer afford this big house or nice car? If the industry takes a dive, and I need to find a new career, then I'm ruined because this is all that I know. Or if I'm an athlete and I'm injured, what value do I have now?

To release suffering, we've got to understand that we are so much more than the things we have, the way we look, the roles we play, the activities we do, and the jobs we have.

In a stripped-down state, we must see that we are so much more than that.

We are eternal beings with ever-expanding consciousness.

The Script:
Lengthen your spine, get comfortable, and settle in.

Close your eyes.

We are going to utilize this meditation to STRIP DOWN.

But first, let's look at all of the ways you describe yourself.

What physical attributes? What personality traits?

What is your astrological sign or your enneagram type?

What is your love language?

What do you do for a living? What role do you play within your work, or are you in between jobs or retired?

What interests do you have?

What physical activities do you do?

How would you describe your diet?

Would you consider yourself rich or poor?

What role do you have in your family or origin?

What role do you have in your current family?

Do you have a lot of friends? A few close ones?

Now that you can see all the ways that you describe yourself, let's start to remove them.

Imagine removing all of these things one by one, layer by layer.

Visualize this as removing layers of thin cloth.

As you remove them one at a time, they billow out into the wind and disappear.

Go beneath the outer layer of appearance, go deeper than the jobs and roles, farther than the characteristics that others have defined you with, or you have associated with yourself.

Remove the labels that may or may not even be true anymore, or perhaps never were.

Think in your mind "I am_____ _____ _____ ."
Fill in your first, middle, and last name.

Say this silently a few times in your mind.

Now remove your last name and say, "I am _____ _____ ."
Fill in your first and middle name.

Repeat silently a few times.

Remove your middle name too.

Now just say, "I am _____ ."
Fill in just your first name.

Repeat a few times.

Remove your first name.

Now just say "I am."

Repeat over and over.

And what's beyond even that?

Who is observing the "I am" statements?

Who listened to the thought?

This is the part of you that is pure awareness, pure consciousness.

The deepest part of you.

Your innermost self. The part of you that is timeless. Connected to all things everywhere.

This core Self is whole and complete, 100% worthy and loveable.

Already.

Always has been.

Always will be.

Right now. Feel the truth of this.

Allow yourself to experience this state of pure BEING for the next ___ minutes *(as long as you've allotted for this portion of the meditation)*.

GUIDING THEM OUT

Utilize the sound of my voice to bring you back to this time and place.

Take some deeper breaths.

Allow your belly to rise with your inhale, and fall with your exhale. Bring your hands to your heart in prayer position.

So, who are you beneath the identification tags, the labels, the roles, the activities, and the objects that you have or don't have?

Hopefully, you've experienced a greater awareness of who you really are in your stripped-down state beneath all of it.

Bow in, recognizing your immense innate value that resides within your deepest core.

FORGIVING

Time: 10-15 minutes

Teachers Note:

I must say that this one can be triggering for some individuals who have unhealed trauma as they may not be ready, willing, able, or in a safe enough mental place to address this topic.

Some ideas: let your students know that you'll be available after meditation should anyone wish to speak with you for help processing emotions, have a counselor or therapist that you can refer individuals to if they would like extra support, and/or give people advance notice that you will be focusing on forgiveness during this meditation so that they can choose to attend or not.

The Script:

When we carry anger, resentment, sadness, or disappointment about things from the past, it's as if we're wearing a backpack filled with rocks.

The person that it weighs down and continues to harm is you.

In this meditation, we will explore releasing that weight with forgiveness, which can bring up some intense thoughts and emotions from past experiences.

At a specific time in this meditation, you will be asked if you would like to forgive someone for something, but please note that it's optional, and you get to choose if you want to, and are ready to.

The offering will be there and it will be your choice.

Let's begin by taking five deep breaths, in through your nose and out through your mouth.

Inhale filling up your belly first, then your chest, exhale let it go.

Two, deep inhale, exhale.

Three, inhale, fully exhale.

Four, slowly inhale, and exhale it out.

Five, inhale, exhale letting it all go.

Allow your breath to return to its normal rhythm.

Bring your awareness to the middle of your breastbone.

Draw a sense of warmth there. Allow it to spread across your chest like warm honey.

Feel this sense of warmth permeate your heart, bringing with it a feeling of comfort and ease.

Connect to the deeper peaceful presence that is within you for a few moments.

(Wait 20 seconds)

Ask if there is something specific that you need to forgive yourself for, whether in your present or from your past.

Something you've been holding against yourself; shame or discomfort that you feel about something.

If you find something there, acknowledge it.

Check to see if there is any deeper understanding or knowledge to be gained from it. If so, receive and integrate the knowledge.

Now, If you're ready, you may choose to forgive yourself and release it. Imagine this dense energy leaving your body like a puff of smoke rising and instantly dissipating into the ether.

Next, ask if there is something that you're ready to forgive someone else for whether in your present or your past.

See if any anger, sadness, disappointment, or resentment comes to your awareness at this time. If something arises, acknowledge it.

Ask if there is any deeper learning or further understanding that you can receive now. If there is, receive and integrate the knowledge.

If you're ready, you may choose to forgive the person, and release any distressful thoughts or emotions connected with it. See it transform into a puff of smoke, instantly dissipating until it's gone.

If there are any tangled thoughts or feelings that you are unworthy or unlovable, you may also choose to release them now.

Every experience, including the difficult and painful ones, has led to your growth and brought you a greater capacity for understanding. Your deepest pain brings with it your greatest gift.

Perhaps it is still unfolding, but every difficulty has a benefit equal to or greater than your suffering.

All of your challenges have served to awaken you, to free you, to help you expand. You may choose to acknowledge and integrate this now.

GUIDING THEM OUT

Take a slow, deep, intentional breath from the bottom to the top of your lungs.

Exhale, release it through your mouth with an audible, "Ahhhhh."

Again, slow deep breath in, and exhale let it go, "Ahhhhh."

Once more, deep breath in, and exhale letting go, "Ahhhhh."

Allow your breathing to return to normal.

Notice how you feel now. Without judgment, just noticing.

Sit up tall, bring your hands to your heart, and pause for a moment of gratitude for all of life's experiences.

FAMILY GRATITUDE MEDITATION

Time: 10-15 minutes

Teacher's Note:

This meditation may be beneficial to offer around the holidays such as Thanksgiving and Christmas (or similar holidays if your residence is outside of the U.S.) and other religious observances that may center around the family.

This is another meditation that can bring up intense emotion, as many individuals have suffered abuse at the hands of their family members.

Those with unhealed trauma may not be ready, willing, able, or in a safe enough mental place to shift to gratitude yet.

Some ideas: Let your students know that you will be available after meditation should anyone wish to speak with you for help processing emotions, and have the name and contact information of a counselor or therapist that you can refer individuals to if they would like extra support.

The Script:

Lengthen your spine, draw your shoulder blades down your back, and open your chest.

Close your eyes. Begin observing your breath for a few cycles.

(wait 30 seconds)

Start to draw your inhale into the lower portion of your lungs, expanding your belly, and exhale allowing your abdomen to relax.

Observe the sensation of the rise and fall of your stomach a few times, listening to the sound of your inhales and exhales as your body releases tension and relaxes.

For this meditation, we are going to focus on gratitude for our family.

Consider first your mother and father. Whether they were in your life or not, they provided life for you.

Give thanks for the gift of life.

Perhaps there were some positive teachings that you have brought with you.

And painful experiences provided an opportunity for you to either choose to follow in their footsteps, or to do something different or opposite.

Your experiences and beliefs that you formed from them have shaped you into the person you are today.

Explore an offering of gratitude for this.

Remember your grandparents on your father's side.

Honor them for the gift of life, whether they were involved in your upbringing or not.

If you did not know them, perhaps you were told stories about them.

Note any special qualities, skills, or insights that you have received from them.

Consider your grandparents on your mother's side.

Whether they were involved in your life or not, give thanks to them for giving your family line life.

What attributes have you gained from their lineage?

What have you learned from them that stands out?

If you have siblings, consider each one with gratitude for the part that they play or played in your life.

Some times were so loving and supportive, other times were challenging. Each of these experiences has taught you something about yourself and about life.

Think of any aunts, uncles, cousins, or extended family that have had special significance in your life.

What stands out to you as you remember your experience with each of them? What did you learn to do or not to do, from them?

Now bring to your awareness those special people who are not related to you by blood, but came into your life and became your chosen family.

These relationships have also expanded your capacity for love, acceptance, and perhaps playfulness or personal growth.

Who comes to mind now?

What do you remember about their special qualities, your experience with them, or what you learned from them?

Every relationship has a special place in your life. Each one is meaningful in some way.

Your life has been enhanced by your connections with them, and even those experiences one would deem negative or painful have brought with them many gifts that have spurred your evolution.

See if there is any new understanding you have received, just by doing this meditation.

(Allow a minute to receive a message.)

GUIDING THEM OUT

Bring your awareness back to your body now and guide some slow deep breaths into your lungs.

Bring your hands together in prayer position at your heart and bow your chin to your chest as a sign of gratitude for all of the people you have journeyed through life with, honoring each of them for who they are, what you experienced together, and their contribution to your life.

MOONLIGHT MEDITATION

Time: 10- 15 minutes

Teacher's Note:
This meditation is wonderful to practice outside at night, or when you'd like to generate cool, calm, and/or magical qualities.

The Script:

Close your eyes and begin to tune inwards. Become aware of the sensations within your body, and notice if you find any places of tension.

We'll take some breaths now, inhaling and exhaling through the nose.

Take a slow, deep breath in through your nose for a count of
1, 2, 3, 4.

Hold your breath for a moment,
then exhale through your nose,
1, 2, 3, 4.

Hold your awareness on the places you feel tension,
Inhale 1, 2, 3, 4.

Allow the tension to release with your exhale,
1, 2, 3, 4.

Inhale into the tension,
1, 2, 3, 4.

Exhale releasing tension,
1, 2, 3, 4.

Check, is there any more residual tightness?

If so, keep your awareness there,
Inhale
1, 2, 3, 4.

Exhale, release it all.
Let it go,
1, 2, 3, 4.

Last one like this,
Inhale
1, 2, 3, 4.

Exhale,
let it all go,
1, 2, 3, 4.

Now breathe smoothly as you allow yourself to feel more comfortable and relaxed.

In this peaceful state, form an image in your mind that you are outside at night.

The air is temperate, and there is a light breeze that dances on your skin. Continue to breathe in and out, feeling the night air gently touch your skin.

Within your mind's eye, you can see the sky in all directions.

The sky is clear, with stars twinkling everywhere.

The moon is full above you. You can hear the steady song of crickets.

Focus on the moon now.

Its light, cool, silvery, and mysterious qualities. Feel the moonlight on your shoulders and your legs.

It feels like the softest embrace.

Allow yourself to soak in its magical, silver light. It's so calming.

How does your body feel under the moonlight?

What is your body temperature like?

How does your heart rate react?

How does your breath respond?

Feel the moonlight on your face and head.

Its soft light reaches down your neck and shoulders, arms and hands, to your fingertips.

The light descends down your torso, thighs, and legs into your toes.

You are now completely bathed in moonlight.

Allow yourself to feel its qualities: cool, calm, soft, gentle.

Maybe the moon or its qualities have something to tell you, some message for you to receive.

We'll be here for a couple of minutes as you continue breathing slowly in and out.

Just be open to receiving and see what appears to you.

(Wait 2 minutes)

GUIDING THEM OUT

Our moon bath is coming to a close now.

When you are ready, take a longer, deeper breath.

Exhale slowly.

Take another deep inhale.

Exhale slowly through your mouth.

Bring your awareness back to this time and place.

Reach your arms above your head and squeeze your muscles, yawning if you like, then open your eyes.

As you exit this meditation, allow the calm, peaceful, luminous qualities of the moon to remain with you.

In appreciation of the moon and all of its beautiful mystery, bow in, chin to chest.

EXISTENTIAL MEDITATION

Time: This meditation can last from 10 - 20 minutes depending on how long you pause between words. You can allow the space in the middle of the meditation to be as short or long as you desire.

Teacher's Note:

Several years ago an eye exam revealed that I had a tear in my retina. After seeing a specialist, I was told that if it rips more, it was possible I'd become blind in the eye. During the same week, I was guided through a meditation similar to this one. I wondered, what if I never see another giraffe, ladybug, butterfly or a hippo again?!!! (I've never been into hippos, but the thought of not being able to see one again was a surprising worry! Haha!)

It was a profound meditation!!! Even though most people won't have the added worry that I had, it's a meditation that usually instills a deep appreciation and reverence for all of the wonderful creations and beauty that we get to experience here on earth (and beyond).

This one is best done while lying down.

The Script:

Lie down on your back for this mediation.

You can place a bolster or pillow underneath your knees if you like, or use an eye mask or blanket for extra comfort. Close your eyes.

Begin by taking some slow, deep breaths. For the next minute, simply observe your breath.

(Wait one minute)

Consider this world that we live in.

The vast tapestry of people, animals, foliage, oceans, landmasses, buildings, and objects. Picture our world within your mind.

(Allow a minute or two to ponder)

Now start removing the buildings from your mental landscape - the skyscrapers, businesses, houses, and apartments.

Next, remove the cars, buses, trains, planes, and bicycles. Take away the animals - insects, mammals, reptiles, and birds.

Take away the people from your internal image. Imagine them popping out of existence.

Remove the forests, deserts, mountains, rocks, bushes, grass, flowers, and cactus.

Take away the boats, the water mammals, fish, and coral reefs.

Take away the bodies of water, the oceans.

Take away the earth itself.

Remove the solar system and star formations.

Remove all of the objects in space.

In this space....FLOAT..... BE.....PURE CONSCIOUSNESS.....PURE AWARENESS.....PURE ENERGY.

(Wait a few minutes)

Bring the stars back into your field of consciousness.

See the recognizable systems of stars and planets.

See a blank earth.

Add the bodies of water and the coral reefs.

The whales, dolphins, and fish.

The continents.

Add mountains, savannas, deserts, and beaches.

The grass, the trees, the flowers.

Animals: lions, hippos, giraffes, butterflies, ladybugs, and lizards.

Add the buildings, businesses, and houses.

Add the modes of transportation.

Bikes, taxis, cars, trains, airplanes.

Add the humans.

(Wait 30 seconds)

GUIDING THEM OUT

Bring your awareness back to your particular body, keeping your eyes closed.

Imagine this is the first time you take a breath.

Breathe in, and let the sensation of oxygen fill your lungs, bringing life to your extremities.

Continue to take nice slow, deep breaths. Imagine this is the first time you are in your body, feeling sensations.

What do you notice in your body?

What sounds do you hear?

What do you smell?

Roll to your side, in the fetal position.

Blink your eyes softly open.

Imagine this is the first time you are seeing out of your eyes.

What colors, shapes, and patterns do you see?

Rise slowly up to a seat and bring your hands to your heart.

Feel your thumbs resting on your breastbone.

Can you feel the beat of your heart?

In Closing:

Perhaps you bring with you a renewed sense of wonder; a new vibrancy, awareness, and appreciation as you re-enter the world.

If your experience was different from that, that's okay too.

What was this meditation like for you?

CONNECTING BODY, MIND, AND SPIRIT

Time: 15 minutes

Teacher's Note:

We generally resist the mind's chatter and proclivity to keep us safe through limiting thoughts. We tend to not want to feel our hearts because it opens us up to vulnerability. And we're often in a state of "doing" or fight or flight, and forget that we are a BEING having an experience on our soul's journey.

This meditation helps us acknowledge, appreciate and connect our mind, heart, and spirit for an optimized human experience.

The Script:
Find a position that is comfortable to you, lengthen your spine, and draw the wingtips of your shoulder blades down your back.

Begin by taking a few slow deep breaths.

Allow your belly to inflate as you inhale, and deflate as you exhale.

Feel your body releasing tension, and let go of any worries and stress, breathing deeply in and out....in and out.

Bring your awareness to the space between your eyebrows.

Instead of looking out with our eyes, we are going to focus inward.

Guide your attention deep into the space behind your eyebrows.

With your inner vision, imagine seeing the electrical impulses firing in your brain. The transportation of information moving through your brain.

Even though your brain may tend to worry, see the beauty of this supercomputer, and thank it for all it does to keep you safe.

Tell your brain that in this present moment everything is okay.

All is good in your world.

As a gift to your mind, send it a beautiful image of a place, or landscape you enjoy.

Someplace you've been or have seen in a picture or a movie. A peaceful place.

Provide as many rich details as you can for the next couple of minutes. What it looks like, what it smells like there, and how the air feels on your skin.

(Wait 1-2 minutes)

Now shift your attention to your chest and the space within your rib cage.

If you notice any tightness there, allow it to dissolve. Arrive at your heart, and sense it like a closed fist, now softly opening.

Feel a warm sensation spreading through your heart and expanding throughout your entire chest. With this comes a feeling of acceptance, wholeness, and love.

Accepting others exactly as they are in this moment.

Accepting yourself exactly as you are in this moment, and accepting the world exactly as it is in this moment.

Allow this feeling to permeate throughout your entire body; this warmth, this love.

Send it down your torso and through your legs all the way to your toes. Across your chest through your arms to your fingertips.

Through your neck into your head all the way to your crown. Feel every cell in your entire body vibrating with this energy.

(Wait for 1-2 minutes)

Notice that there is a part of you that's been listening to these guiding words.

The you that is watching yourself.

Watching your brain thinking these images and witnessing these sensations.

 This is the infinite, inner being that is who you really are beneath your outward identity. This part of you is peaceful, understanding, light, and expansive.

Feel its connection to your heart and mind.

Feel the energy flow between your body, your mind, and your heart, making the connection stronger and more balanced.

With this higher-self connection, your thoughts have a broader perspective, your heart has deeper feelings, and your body sends messages as signals, felt throughout.

A synergistic symphony.

Recognize the beauty of the connection, and allow yourself to bask in the harmony of balance and cohesion here for a few minutes.

(Wait 2-3 minutes)

GUIDING THEM OUT

Slowly bring your awareness back.

Stretch your body, reach your arms above your head, yawn, and squeeze your muscles.

Appreciate the sensations that you feel.

If you're feeling out of balance sometime in the future, remember that you can do this again.

 It is now a tool in your toolbox.

Tune into your mind, your heart, and your true, expansive, infinite self.

With balance, you now re-enter the world as one cohesive self.

ASCENDING CHAKRA ACTIVATION MEDITATION

Time: About 15 minutes, or longer if you wish to add silence at the end.

Teacher's note:

This meditation offers a sequential journey through the seven main chakras, activating and balancing them through intentional awareness.

Sometimes we overcomplicate things, and easier is better ;).

We'll put our highest selves in charge to help us make the necessary adjustments.

This one is best done while seated.

The Script:

This meditation will help rebalance your chakras.

It's best practiced while seated so that the chakras align vertically.

Feel free to use a yoga block, bolster, or cushion underneath you, or even sit against a wall if you feel that you need extra support to hold your body in this position.

Lift your spine nice and tall, with a slight engagement of your core to assist your posture.

Close your eyes.

We'll begin with three deep breaths, in through your nose and out through your mouth.

Inhale through your nose, and exhale, open mouth, making a "haaaaa" sound.

Inhale nose, exhale mouth.

Again.

Now take seven more breaths, this time with lips sealed, breathing in and out of your nose only.

(Guide or count seven more breaths)

We are going to put your highest self in charge, your wisdom self, your superconscious, asking for assistance to create the necessary adjustments that allow your chakras to balance with gentleness and ease.

We are energetic, quantum beings. When we make a change energetically, our entire system responds instantly.

Energy is without bounds of time, so we can go directly to the place where it can be changed immediately. Choose this understanding now.

Visualize yourself sitting in a place that is peaceful to you.

If you feel challenged visualizing, just imagine that you can, as if you're watching a movie of yourself.

This could be a place in nature or an indoor space that is beautiful and serene. Add a few more details to the setting now.

For this meditation, we'll be employing a golden thread of energy to light up and balance each of our 7 major chakras, one by one, starting with the Root.

Whatever scene you've found yourself in, imagine that you are sitting down cross-legged, and a bright, golden light appears beneath you.

This golden light activates your Root Chakra. At the base of your torso the color red appears, glowing vibrantly.

As the energy center rebalances, you become more grounded, stable, and secure, feeling that you belong.

Next, the golden light travels a little higher to your second chakra, the Sacral Chakra. In between the base of your spine and navel, a bright, glowing orange color becomes visible, connecting you with your creativity and emotions.

Notice what emotion is present for you now.

The gold light travels higher to your third chakra, your Solar Plexus Chakra. A bright yellow light like the sun emerges within the area between your navel and your chest, activating your sense of internal power and self-trust.

Now the light arrives at the fourth chakra at the center of your chest, your Heart Chakra. An emerald green light illuminates the area. You feel pure love radiating from the energy center, expansive and warm.

The golden light moves higher to your neck, activating your Throat Chakra with the color blue. An electric blue light reveals itself, unblocking stagnation, and allowing you to express yourself and communicate kindly and clearly.

The light enters the space between your eyebrows, your Third Eye Chakra. A bright bluish-purple color appears, rebooting your inner guidance system, allowing you to see things more clearly and receive messages from your highest self.

The golden light travels to the very top of your head, your Crown Chakra. A brilliant white light illuminates the area, showing you how you are connected to everything in the universe.

Experiencing this unicity, a wave of peace and energy washes over you from head to toe.

Now that your energy centers are fully activated and re-balanced, feel how alive your entire system feels. How harmonic, and congruent you feel.

Bask here in this state of BEING for the next _____ minutes (however long you have allotted for this meditation).

GUIDING THEM OUT

Bring your awareness back to your breath. Inhale, feel your belly rise; exhale, feel your belly fall.

Again, great big inhale; and exhale, and let it go.

Open your eyes as you bring your hands to your chest in prayer position, bowing in to appreciate the attunement of all of the incredible energy that exists within you.

CHAKRA BALANCING MEDITATION

Time: About 15-20 minutes

Teacher's Note:

There is such abundant information about chakras out there, that diving in can easily become overly complicated.

This Chakra Meditation is straightforward, distilled down to the main expression of the energy balance/imbalance, and provides a big impact.

There is an affirmation listed for each chakra that can be repeated out loud or silently to optimize and balance the energy there, as well as an associated Bija Mantra. "Bija" means seed. These are single syllables that when chanted, balance the energy and bring harmony to the chakra. You could use these instead of the affirmations if you like, or for a lengthier meditation, use both.

You may wish to focus on just one chakra for the entire meditation or move through each of them.

The Script:

This meditation is best practiced seated so that your chakras are aligned vertically.

However, if sitting doesn't work for your body at this time, feel free to lie down.

If you are seated, you can utilize a yoga block, bolster, or cushion underneath you for support.

Lift your spine nice and tall, with a slight engagement of your core to assist your elevated posture. Close your eyes.

Let's begin by bringing awareness to the 1st Chakra:
The Root Chakra, located at the base of your spine.
The color of this chakra is red.

Imagine the color red glowing at the root of your torso.

It's the place of survival, security, and safety. It pertains to your relationship with your family of origin and animal instincts.

It's imbalanced by fear. Exhale, release fear; inhale, a sense of safety. Exhale, release fear; inhale, a sense of safety.

Affirmation: "I am safe and secure. I have everything that I need."
Repeat three times, if using the affirmation.

Bija Mantra: Lam (pronounced like Lum, rhymes with thumb) *Repeat three times, if using the bija mantra.*

Now let's shift our attention to the 2nd Chakra:
The Sacral Chakra, between your navel and pubic bone.
The color is orange.

Imagine the color orange glowing within your lower abdomen.

It houses your sexuality, creativity, joy, and your relationship with abundance/money.

It's imbalanced by guilt. Exhale, release guilt; inhale, a sense of pleasure and joy.

Exhale, release guilt; inhale, feel the abundance that already exists within you.

Affirmation: "I allow myself the freedom to experience pleasure and joy. I live in absolute abundance." *Repeat three times, if using the affirmation.*

Bija Mantra: Vam (pronounced like Vum, rhymes with thumb). *Repeat three times, if using the bija mantra.*

Guide your awareness a little higher up now to the 3rd Chakra: The Solar Plexus Chakra, located between the navel and chest. The color is yellow.

Imagine the color yellow glowing at the center of your torso.

It deals with willpower, self-confidence, and your ability to manifest.

It's imbalanced by shame.

Exhale, release shame; inhale, bravery.

Exhale, release shame; inhale, and feel the power and strength of will at your center.

Affirmation: "I accept myself completely, and I create my life the way I want it." *Repeat three times, if using the affirmation.*

Bija Mantra: Ram (pronounced like rum). *Repeat three times, if using the bija mantra.*

Let's travel to the 4th Chakra: The Heart Chakra, positioned in the middle of your chest. The color is green.

Imagine the color emerald green glowing at the center of your chest.

It deals with love, forgiveness, hope, and compassion. It's imbalanced by grief.

Exhale, release grief; inhale a sense of being loved.

Exhale, release grief; inhale a sense of giving love to others.

Affirmation: "It's easy for me to give and receive love, because I am love." *Repeat three times, if using the affirmation.*

Bija Mantra: Yam (pronounced like Yum, rhymes with thumb). *Repeat three times, if using the bija mantra.*

Shift your awareness now to the 5th Chakra: The Throat Chakra.
The color is blue.

Imagine a blue light glowing within your throat.

This is where you hold truth, communication, and self-expression.

It's blocked by lies.

Exhale the need to omit or alter information;
inhale the strength to give and receive the truth.

Exhale, release timidness;
inhale the strength to express who you really are.

Affirmation: "It's easy for me to communicate and express myself."
Repeat three times, if using the affirmation.

Bija Mantra: Ham (pronounced like hum).
Repeat three times, if using the bija mantra.

Guide your focus to the 6th Chakra: The Third Eye Chakra, located in the center of your eyebrows, lining up with the pineal gland. The color is indigo.

Imagine a brilliant purplish-blue light glowing between your brows.

It deals with insight, intuition, visualization, perception, and psychic awareness.

It is blocked by illusion.

Exhale, release the veils of illusion;
inhale greater insight.

Exhale, release mental congestion;
inhale clarity.

Affirmation: "I see with clarity, and I trust my intuition." *Repeat three times, if using the affirmation.*

Bija Mantra: Om. *Repeat three times, if using the bija mantra.*

And lastly, let's journey to the 7th Chakra: The Crown Chakra, located on top of the head.

It's the spiritual center, housing pure universal energy, enlightenment, unity, and is blocked by earthly attachments and singularity.

The color is white.

Imagine a brilliant white light glowing at the top of your head.

Exhale, release attachment to objects;
inhale pure energy, healing and energizing.

Exhale, release feelings of isolation;
inhale, remember that you are connected to everything and everyone,
a part of the energy of ALL THAT IS.

Affirmation: "I AM." *Repeat three times, if using the affirmation.*

Bija Mantra: Om. *Repeat three times, if using the bija mantra.*

GUIDING THEM OUT

Keeping your eyes closed, check in with yourself and notice if any of these chakras were easier or more challenging to connect with energetically or visually.

In this way, you may be able to identify imbalances and can look up various methods to bring balance back to the specific energy centers that need a little more love and attention.

When you are ready, open your eyes.

If you are lying down, bend your knees and slowly roll to one side, then help yourself up to a seated position.

Draw your hands to your chest and bow in.

Namaste.

LET GO, GIVE THANKS, & CALL IN

Time: 20 minutes. Longer if you'd like time to rest in silence afterward.

Teacher's Note:

I love offering this one around Thanksgiving or Christmas, because it's a beautiful time to give thanks, (and maybe because of the movies we watch as a family like Harry Potter or The Lord of the Rings :), there's a quality to the season that inspires thoughts of ancient magic, grassy hills, and old stone castles.

For those who live outside of the U.S., perhaps there's another holiday or time of the year that this meditation fits well within.

This one is best done while lying down, but you can adjust the language if your setting requires meditators to be seated.

The Script:

Lie down on your back.

Get comfortable.

Feel free to place a pillow underneath your head, your knees, and a blanket over you if you like.

Close your eyes.

Guide some slow, deep breaths into your lower belly.

Imagine you're walking on a beautiful green, grassy hillside like the moors of Scotland.

As you look down a hill, you see a big stone castle in the area below. You feel drawn to walk down towards it.

As you get closer, you see giant, 30-foot, red, double doors that are open. You decide to walk through them onto the cool stone floor.

You look to the left and notice stairs that curl up and around to the floor above.

You begin to walk up the stone steps.

You see your right foot step up, then your left, 3, 4, 5, the smell is a bit musty, 6, 7, 8, 9, 10.

You hear the crackle before you see it.

As you step out into an open space you notice a large, ornate fire pit in the middle of the room with a robust fire going.

As you look around, you see ornate tapestries on the walls and big rectangular windows without panes.

Long draperies frame them in jewel tones of emerald, ruby, and sapphire, billowing in the breeze.

You walk over to the fire pit and stare at the burning logs and glowing embers.

The orange and yellow flames dance.

You feel the warmth that emanates from it and hear the popping sparks.

You know intrinsically that you are meant to leave something behind in this fire.

Some quality or habit that no longer serves you, perhaps a negative thought or emotion, even a physical pain, or symptom of ill health.

Imagine reaching inside of your metaphysical self with your right hand, drawing it out of you.

Once you pull it out, place it in your left hand.

Then go in again with your right hand one more time and make sure that you have all of it.

Transfer any remnants into your left hand, and place your right hand underneath your left.

Look at what you hold in your hands. It may be slightly gray or darkened.

Look at it and give thanks for any purpose that it served in your life, whether known or unknown.

Now place it in the fire. It sizzles when you put it in, and ignites. Bright sparks shoot up about 3ft above the rim. It combusts into a million particles of bright light that instantly return to the ether.

You may notice that you feel lighter and freer, unburdened.

You hadn't noticed how much it had weighed you down because you'd gotten used to it.

But now that you've released it you can breathe so much easier. Now that it's gone you feel so much better. It's surprising really.

You find yourself drawn to the right side of the room now and start walking in that direction.

You see a low, small, square, light brown wooden table.

On the table sits two candles and some long matches in a matchbox.

One candle is white and one is yellow.

Beneath the table is a beautiful turquoise floor pillow with golden embellishments and tassels.

You kneel or sit on the pillow in front of the candles.

You have an inner knowing that guides your attention to the white candle first. Here you are meant to thank your ancestors.

You use a match to light the white candle in honor of your mother and father (perhaps you had more than one) whether they were in your life or not, your grandparents, and great-grandparents.

You may have been raised by another family member or had some other influential guides in your life that you wish to focus on or include.

Whether positive or negative, what was passed down from them helped shape who you are now. Give thanks and honor each of them.

You may even choose to ask if there is a message for you to receive from any of them at this time.

Once this feels complete, you blow out the white candle and watch the trail of smoke drift upwards toward the high ceiling.

Now you shift your attention to the yellow candle and light it.

You watch the flame flicker and then stabilize.

With this candle you are meant to call something into your life: a new job or relationship, a new personal quality or positive habit to support you in some way, vibrant health, prosperity, enhanced intuition, or another spiritual gift,.. whatever it is that you believe you are ready to receive.

Choose something powerful, and say it in a sentence:
"I am now calling _____into my life."

You may see some images about this come into your mind. You may see a vision of yourself doing something now that you have it.

If so, notice who you're with, what the setting is, what it smells and tastes like there, and most importantly, HOW YOU FEEL.

Allow the details to fill in so fully and richly that it seems that it is already happening.

When this feels complete, gaze at the yellow candle again, and watch how the flame glows brighter and bigger for a moment.

Then blow it out.

GUIDING THEM OUT

Your time here is soon coming to a close, but you know that you can come here whenever you wish.

Next time you come, you can add your own alters, rooms, and experiences. You can decorate it however you wish.

The setting can morph and change as you do. For now, rise up from the pillow, take one last look around the room, and head towards the stairs.

Starting at ten, step one foot down, 9, the other foot down, 8, keep going nice and slow 7, 6, 5, feel the cool, concrete wall to the side, 4, 3, 2, 1, finding yourself facing the giant, open, red double doors.

You walk out into the sunlight onto the soft emerald-green grass.

Smell the fresh air.

You are ready to return to your physical body now.

This magical place dissipates into a million particles of golden light and you find yourself lying on your back in this time and place. Feel the floor beneath you.

Take several slow, deep, belly breaths.

Wiggle your fingers and toes.

Welcome back.

Gently roll onto your right side, and use your left hand to guide yourself into your favorite seated posture.

Guide your hands to the center of your chest.

Namaste.

5 KOSHAS MEDITATION

Time: about 35 minutes, or you can break it up into 5 shorter meditations and explore them separately

---

Teacher's Note:

This meditation offers a journey into each of the layers of self as outlined by the ancient Vedic text, the Taittiriya Upanishad.

Each of these layers, called koshas, can be explored as its own mini-meditation if you wish to break this up into smaller components.

For example, if you're using it for a yoga class, each week you could focus on a different kosha. For a comprehensive experience, guide it in its entirety.

The Script:

The Koshas are the energetic "sheaths" or layers that make up our whole self, first described in an ancient Vedic text called the Taittiriya Upanishad written around the sixth century B.C.

From our deep spiritual core to our outermost layer of skin, they are our physical body, breath/lifeforce, mental body, wisdom body, and bliss body/soul.

Focusing on your koshas helps you develop a stronger connection between your body, mind, and spirit, allowing you to experience deeper states of awareness and a greater understanding of your True Self.

For the first two koshas, you will be seated, and for the last three, you will be lying down.

To start, place your bolster or cushion underneath you if you would like to use one, and sit up tall.

Rest your palms facing down on your thighs, enabling you to turn your attention inwards.

Start by bringing awareness to your PHYSICAL BODY.
The ANNAMAYA KOSHA.

Activate your root lock, Mula Bandha, by lifting and engaging your pelvic floor muscles. This provides anchoring and grounding.

Next, activate Uddiyana Bandha, your belly lock, by drawing your navel back towards your spine, stabilizing the energy at your core center.

Then squeeze the muscles around your heart.

Both the front of the heart, firming the muscles of your chest, and the back of the heart, hugging your shoulder blades in.

Activate awareness at your heart center by giving the surrounding muscles a little squeeze.

Gently release the muscle engagement now and just notice your skin.

Notice the places where you are touching the ground or where your hands touch your legs. Notice the air on your skin.

Feel the outer layer of your body.

Now we'll shift to the PRANAMAYA KOSHA which houses our BREATH/LIFEFORCE.

Become aware of your body breathing. Notice the subtle energetic flow of sensation and feeling as you breathe.

Sense oxygen filling your lungs, entering your bloodstream, bringing aliveness to your physical body and mind.

Your exhale expelling carbon dioxide. Try not to figure anything out, just experience the sensation.

The sensations that the inhales evoke within you, and the sensations that come with the exhales.

I'll count down 10 cycles of breath from 10 down to 1. *(Guide each inhale and exhale slowly and evenly, at about a 5-count).*

Inhale 10, Exhale 10

Inhale 9, Exhale 9

Inhale 8, Exhale 8

Inhale 7, Exhale 7

Inhale 6, Exhale 6

Inhale 5, Exhale 5

Inhale 4, Exhale 4

Inhale 3, Exhale 3

Inhale 2, Exhale 2

Inhale 1, Exhale 1

Now come back to the awareness of your body breathing itself.
(Allow about 1 minute here)

Make your way onto your back now. If you have a pillow or a bolster, you may want to place it underneath your knees for added support and comfort.

Close your eyes.

We will next explore the MANOMAYA KOSHA, your FEELINGS and EMOTIONS.

We will explore polarities, starting with ANXIETY VS. CALM

Remember a time this week or month when you felt anxious.

Maybe your body felt racy, or you felt your heart pounding or tension in your stomach or head.

Go back to what that experience was like.

Notice where you feel it the most.

LET IT GO. COME BACK TO NEUTRAL

Now consider the time this week or this month that you felt the most peaceful and calm.

What does that feel like in your system?

What do you notice?

Perhaps it's even an absence of a feeling, an openness.

SAD VS. JOYFUL

Think of a time when you were sad recently.

Maybe due to something going on in your life, something going on with a friend or someone you care about, or something going on in the world.

Where is this feeling concentrated the most?

What does it feel like?

LET IT GO, AND COME BACK TO NEUTRAL

Now shift to some time in the last week or month that you felt very happy, joyful, or even elated.

Maybe something good happened in your life, or you heard some good news from a friend or loved one and you felt so happy for them.

What sensations come up in your body?

Where do you feel it?

HEAVY VS. LIGHT

Next, feel the sensation of heaviness within your body.

Your back sinking into the earth, your legs, heavy like lead resting on the ground.

Your shoulders feel weighted. Y

our head sinks lower into your mat.

Your eyes rest in their sockets.

Allow yourself to feel the sensation of gravity.

Rooted, weighted.

LET IT GO, AND COME BACK TO NEUTRAL.

Now bring a sense of lightness into your body.

Chest and heart open, relaxed, and light. Belly expansive.

Arms and legs feel so light that they might start floating.

Jaw totally relaxed. Cheekbones tingle, forehead lighter.

The Crown of your head is open, your body getting lighter as if it'll start levitating up.

LET IT GO, AND COME BACK TO NEUTRAL.

(Allow some time ~15-30 seconds)

Next up is VIJNANAMAYA KOSHA - the INSIGHT layer.

If there has been a question on your mind lately, a decision you need to make, or a challenge you have been facing, bring it to mind now.

If there's nothing like this that you've been experiencing lately, then just remain open and see what messages you receive.

We'll be tapping into our insight layer by asking some questions.

Just allow yourself to be open to receiving the information that your wisdom self wishes to relay.

What is it that I need to see? *(Wait 15 seconds.)*

What is it that I need to hear? *(Wait 15 seconds.)*

What is it that I need to know?*(Wait 15 seconds.)*

What needs to shift in my life for this to happen?*(Wait 15 seconds.)*

What condition can I adjust to make this a reality?*(Wait 15 seconds.)*

Perhaps you have received a bit of wisdom from your insight layer.

(Wait 15-30 seconds.)

Finally, the ANANDAMAYA KOSHA - BLISS

This is where we allow all sensations, breath, feelings, and thoughts to be present, just as they are.

Notice that throughout all of these practices, you have been observing and witnessing the experiences.

Allow this sense of awareness to permeate.

The spacious presence of awareness.

BEING spacious presence......being spacious presence.

Pure awareness.

Pure consciousness.

Tingly and alive.

Open and Expansive.

A pure state of BEING that may feel like bliss.

(Wait 30 seconds).

GUIDING THEM OUT

Take a moment to walk back through this journey that we've just taken.

Breathing, feeling sensations in the body, experiencing emotion, thoughts coming and going, insights discovered.

Witnessing all of it. All of these things make up your whole self.

Gently roll to one side, open your eyes, and help yourself back up to a seated posture.

As we close, consider the totality of your being.

The presence of spacious awareness at your core, the energy that runs through you, the emotions and sensations that are expressed through you, and the thoughts that help inform you.

Feel the magic of this entirety.

The entirety of YOU.

Bring your hands to your heart center,

Namaste.

WISDOM BYTES

Food for thought & inpsiration that can be
offered for students to consider at the end of
a yoga or meditation class before they re-
enter the world again.

Feel free to use these in your newsletters,
emails, and social media posts as well, with
author credit "Kelli Russell".

AND NOW WE BEGIN

And now we begin. We start at the point that we're at right now.

Even if we feel uneasy, out of balance, weak, or unwell, then that's where we start.

There is no completion, no endpoint to arrive at.

There is just the unfolding. An endless BECOMING.

As we expand into new territory, outside of previously laid boundaries, we become beginners yet again.

So the question is, "Can we bravely step into this endless new adventure?"

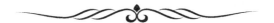

THE ELECTRIC PRESENT

THERE IS SOMETHING POWERFUL TAKING PLACE.

THE ELECTRICITY OF THE PRESENT MOMENT.

HERE....HERE....HERE....IT'S HAPPENING.

At this very moment, there is a totality happening. A state of hereness, a nowness. Connect to this moment. Be in this moment.

Remain in this ever-changing moment. *The electric present.*

CYCLES

There is a cycle that all things in nature, including us, experience: Creation, Homeostasis, Dissolution, and Space before the next creation.

We see this cycle everywhere in nature, in relationships, within our personal development, projects, and businesses.

All organisms, including ourselves, experience it many times in our lives.

But sometimes when something has run its course, we're reluctant to let it go.

And we can become miserable in the dissolution and space because we can't yet see beyond it.

Going around the cycle isn't optional, so pan out.

Draw your perspective outside of it so that you can see it for what it is: the breakdown before the next breakthrough to a new level of evolution and expansion.

Release resistance and recognize that beyond the place you're at right now is your next new beginning.

ASKING BETTER QUESTIONS

Our brains love to plan and protect, and many of the questions we ask ourselves are limiting. Why do I keep messing up? Why is this so hard? Why can't I find a partner? Why can I never get ahead?

Since our minds love to answer questions, why not give our mind better questions, so that we can receive better answers? *For example, ask yourself,*

What can I do today to experience more joy?

How am I so lucky to have deep friendships with amazing people?

How does money keep coming to me in unexpected ways?

How am I becoming more sexy, vibrant, and energetic every day?

What is a possible solution here?

GRATITUDE

If you're stuck in a funk or trapped in a negative loop, take a pause and sincerely give thanks for one thing you feel grateful for.

You will find that a state of expansion like gratitude and a state of contraction cannot exist at the same time.

Notice how easy it is to change your inner state to one of appreciation simply by shifting your attention.

Even better, do something nice for someone else and notice what that does to your inner state :)

TRUST

Trust that with everything that happens, your internal growth, and capacity for understanding will be equal to or greater than the pain you experience.

INSIDE ANSWERS

You'll find many of the answers to the questions you're seeking if you get quiet enough to hear.

Find a quiet spot and get still within your body and mind. Take a few deep breaths, ask your highest self the question, and wait for a few minutes to receive an answer.

The answer may appear as words or an inner knowing, or may arrive in an unexpected way as a symbol, a song lyric, or a feeling.

Be open to what you receive, and if nothing comes through within a few minutes, don't worry.

Remain open and observant; often the answer will appear within the next week or two.

EVOKING PEACE

Knowing that I am in continual growth and evolution,

I accept myself today exactly as I am,

with all of my uniqueness and idiosyncrasies.

And I do the same for others, without judgment,

for I never truly know what they are experiencing.

By doing these things, I am at peace.

INSPIRATIONS

These can be used as meditations, or food for thought to share in classes, workshops, or events.

Also, feel free to share them in your newsletters, emails, and social posts with author credit: "Kelli Russell".

NON-ATTACHED

Life is messy and unpredictable.

Sometimes we have long stretches of peace, success, and love. Sometimes we seem to experience a string of troubles.

We have ups and downs and all arounds. We have periods of productivity and creation and days that are low energy and lethargic.

We sometimes get injured. We sometimes get sick. It's natural to move in and out of balance.

True peace of mind comes from not attaching a great deal of importance to any particular state.

Accepting it all as the natural flow of life.

NOT FORWARD, BUT INWARD

So many of us on the spiritual path to enlightenment expect it to elevate us; that the skills we accumulate will allow us to become something better than we were before.

What a surprise it is to discover that the journey doesn't take us forward, but INWARD.

And it's not about gathering things, it's about letting them go.

We realize that there was nothing that we needed to aspire to or strive for. It is simply uncovering the truth of what was there all along.

EXPANDING AWARENESS

Release the goal of getting rid of your thoughts.

Instead, become MORE aware of them, and allow them to drift through your field of awareness without getting stuck.

Practice observing the thoughts in your mind just as you would see data processing on a screen or graffiti on a wall.

You may find that it's just chatter, and some, if not most of it, is inconsequential and repetitive.

Its job is mostly planning and protecting.

Your mind is an organ working for you like your lungs are breathing and your heart is beating.

You will soon realize that you are not your thoughts, you are the WATCHER of your thoughts, THE OBSERVER.

In this way, you remember your soulful self, and your thoughts lose their power.

Now ask yourself, "What is beyond this mental chatter?

What's deeper than this?"

You may be surprised by what you find...

ANCHORED IN CALMNESS

Begin to notice the rhythm of your breath. Slow it down.

Let calmness infuse you.

As you take your next breath, amplify this calmness.

Feel how quiet it is.

Amplify this quietness until it permeates all of your senses.

Feel anchored in your calmness no matter what is going on around you.

Feel it in the soles of your feet, your belly, your heart, your hands, and your head.

Grounded in your calmness.

Anchored in the knowing that you can handle anything life brings to you.

STRIPPED DOWN

Take off competition and comparison

Remove guilt,

Shame,

Fear,

Anxiousness,

Sorrow,

Worry,

Timidness,

Resentment,

Judgment,

Someone else's skewed perception of you,

Your own skewed perception of you,

The roles that you play,

The labels that you apply to yourself,

The stress and trauma that you've experienced,

Your story. What is left underneath?

Pure awareness. Pure Consciousness. Pure love. Pure YOU.

JUST A MINUTE

Consider this. It takes just a minute to imagine something you enjoy and your whole body feels light and free.

And it takes just a minute to think of yourself as a failure that no one likes and your shoulders collapse as you feel sorry for yourself.

It takes just a minute to decide to let go of resentment and laugh it off. It takes just a minute to stop judging and see the beauty that is all around you.

Who is doing all of these things? YOU!

Has anything around you changed in the outside world? No!

If you spend your time thinking about all the things that are wrong in your life, you will have a life of misery.

If you often think of things that bring you joy and happiness, then joy and happiness will be yours.

Your thoughts become your reality.

OBSERVING THOUGHTS

Unchecked thoughts dominate our minds and our lives.

We get lost in plans, judgments, and memories.

Many thoughts are fear-based, and most are not even true.

When we get still and really investigate our thoughts, we realize that they're little more than nothing; ephemeral wisps.

Becoming aware of a thought is like waking up from a dream.

We awaken to the movie of our minds.

We shift from being lost in thought to being aware that we are thinking.

Then we are no longer bound by them.

They are no longer our identity.

From the perspective of the observer, we gain a sense of space, peace, and inner calmness.

LIVING FROM YOUR BIG SELF

Have you ever heard the concept of living from your Small Self vs. living from your Big Self?

When you're living from your Small Self, you're contracted, doubting, worrying, fearful, insecure, and judgmental.

When you're living from your Big Self, you're expansive, present, accepting, open, welcoming, easy-going, and vibrant.

Use these words when you need a reminder to live from your Big Self:

"I am open and at peace. I am infinite and expansive. I am part of the energy of ALL THAT IS."

LUMINOSITY ITSELF

YOU ARE an energetic being of great magnitude with consciousness beyond your story.

You are more than the words on the page that make up the story of your life.

You are more than the pages that make up your book. You are more than the binding of your book.

You are more than the space between the pages. You are more than the stories found within the pages.

You are more than the happys and the sads, the goods, and the bads.

You are made of particles and waves.

You are energy at its purest. Pure energy, pure light, pure love.

YOU ARE A RADIANT BEING.

YOU ARE LUMINOSITY ITSELF.

DREAMLIKE LIFE

With a beginner's mind, I see clearly again.

As I release past perceptions weighing me down, I am no longer trapped, constricted, or contained.

My old story begins to lose its hold.

JOY, EASE, and PEACE AWAKEN.

Who do I choose to be now?

What new adventures will commence?

I decide to greet life with a relaxed smile on my face as I remind myself of who I truly am.

An extension of source.

More than my physical body.

More than my 5 senses.

I am connected to ALL THAT IS through higher consciousness.

I realize that I am the creator of my inner world and that my outer experience is simply a reflection.

And the more I realize that my life is but a beautiful lucid dream, The more dreamlike my life becomes.

REMEMBERING

Take a deep breath.

Rinse yourself clean of those old stories you continue to tell about yourself and your life.

You can't go back to the way things were. There's nothing there for you anymore.

But you can BE HERE NOW. You can breathe, and feel, and experience. You can release pent-up energy that some call stress or anxiety. And you can remember.

You can experience a remembering that you are whole and immeasurably valuable exactly as you are.

That things are unfolding perfectly, in perfect timing.

That you have everything you need inside of yourself to be the person that you want to be.

Feel your innate power and the energy that enlivens you, the breath that flows through you.

Feel the peaceful presence that guides you and connects you to everything, everywhere.

What a beautiful, magical remembering.

RELEASE THE PAST

I now choose to release the past.

I am ready to let go of old emotions, thoughts, and patterns
that have had me locked in their hold.

However challenging or difficult some things have been,
however wonderful or enlightening,

I release the familiarity of what was known.

I am ready to leap into the undefined, unexplored, mystery of the
unknown.

Because I now recognize that whether we resist it or not,
expansion occurs.

I am not who I was before,
nor are those around me.

And I am now willing to be less fearful and rigid.

To learn and experiment.

To do what I've never done before.
To experience even more than I imagined.

A leap of faith is what it takes.

I appreciate and thank what was, and welcome the new.

To this ever-unfolding present moment, I surrender.

GO YOUR OWN WAY

We mistakenly believe that there is some "correct" or "right" path that we have to take in life. We take on ideas from our family members, friends, colleagues, and bosses.

We get caught in a trap of perceived obligations and "shoulds" which inhibit our own expression.

However, their ideas and perceptions are not there to establish your path. Their ideas and perceptions are there to establish their path.

To truly live an authentic, fully expressed life, each individual must forge their own way and experience life with their unique viewpoint, skills, interests, likes, and dislikes.

Therefore, It will never suit you to compare yourself to others. And it will never work to convince others that they must think and behave the way you do!

You need to DO YOU, and they need to do them!

Take ownership of your own experience and know what it is to live fully and deeply from your own truth.

Allow others to do the same and you will experience a massive shift in ease, acceptance, and letting go.

A life more finely tuned to joy.

RELEASE RESISTANCE TO EXPERIENCE PEACE

Many of us try to control the uncontrollable by creating an idea of how things are "supposed" to go or be which provides a false sense of security and predictability.

When the unwanted happens, instead of rolling with it, we say, "How can this happen to me?! Why me?!"

We internalize the experience and think the world is conspiring against us.

We shore up our defenses and build walls of protection around ourselves.

These walls may have provided great protection at some point, but now they block our feelings, our soul's expansion, and our connection to others.

When we block our feelings and we're in protection mode, our body gives us warning signals in the form of physical pain, weakness, and even illness.

So how do we release these walls of defense?

We've got to fully accept that life is up and down and all around.

Sometimes things go this way and sometimes things go that way.

We can acknowledge our emotions as the messengers that they are.

Accept all of the experiences this world has to offer with as much gentleness and humor as we can.

Remain OPEN, OBSERVING, and FLEXIBLE, which builds RESILIENCE.

And although we cannot control others or mother nature, we can trust our inner guidance systems (our gut feelings; intuition) to steer us right.

Soon we will get so good at practicing these things, that we can BE in the world without our guard up.

By releasing resistance, we experience newfound peace.

BREATHING PRACTICES

Focused breathing is one of the easiest ways to decrease stress and anxiety and shift into a calm, focused state, changing your chemistry in seconds. If you've studied Bruce Lipton's work in Epigenetics, notably his book *The Biology of Belief*, you've learned that your inner perception of your outer environment can even dictate which genes turn on and off. We can actually change our biology by lessening our stress response! And one of the best ways to shift out of stress and into a state of calm, peaceful presence is through breathwork practices.

In addition to decreasing stress, the breathing practices within this book are designed to enhance circulation, increase blood oxygenation, expand lung capacity, increase focus and awareness, and support your holistic well-being.

MEDICAL DISCLAIMER & CONTRAINDICATIONS FOR BREATHWORK

Teacher's Note: You may wish to share this disclaimer before guiding breathwork.

Breathwork can result in strong emotional and physical responses. Some breathwork is not safe under certain medical conditions such as epilepsy or seizures.

Before practicing breathwork, ask your doctor if there are certain types of breathing practices you should not be practicing, to ensure that you are cleared to do so.

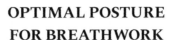

OPTIMAL POSTURE
FOR BREATHWORK

For these breathing techniques, you will either be lying down or sitting up tall.

If you are lying on your back, you may find it more comfortable to place a pillow or bolster under your knees.

If you're sitting, any seated posture is great, as long as your spine is long, your chest is lifted, and your knees, feet, and ankles are comfortable.

For some, sitting cross-legged or in lotus pose will work. Others may prefer bending their knees, sitting on their feet with hips over heels, a.k.a. the thunderbolt pose.

With any seated posture, a cushion or yoga block placed underneath your sitting bones may increase your comfort.

Try out different positions and see which feels best for you. If at any time you feel you need to adjust your posture or change positions, please do.

BOAT BREATH

Time: 3-5 minutes

Teacher's Note:
I like to use this one every now and then at the start of yoga classes followed by some gentle variations of salabhasana/locust pose alternating lifting left leg and right arm, looking left, with lifting right leg and left arm, looking right.

It can also be used within a breathwork practice.

It offers unique biofeedback, because one can feel their belly pressing into the floor with diaphragmatic breathing, ensuring that they're guiding their breath into their belly rather than using the shallow chest breathing that many of us have been accustomed to while in chronic state of stress.

The Script:
Lie down on your belly.

You can place your hands underneath your chin, palms flat, with your nose facing down, or choose to turn your face to one side, resting on your ear.

Imagine that your body is a boat, floating on a sea of energy, of prana. As you inhale, expand your abdomen. Exhale, and at the end of your exhale, draw your navel lightly up towards your spine.

Inhale, and expand your belly.

Exhale all of your breath out, and gently contract your belly.

Continue to inhale and exhale in this way.

Notice that the contraction and expansion create a rise and fall sensation... your boat gently rocking on an energetic sea.

Continue to breathe in this way for the next minute *(or two)*.

Maintain a connection to the rising and falling sensations you're experiencing as you breathe.

Tune in to the subtle waves of energy for the next ___ minutes. *(however long you've allotted for this breathing practice)*

If guiding this breath within a yoga class, at this point you may wish to do some alternate limb salabhasana flow as described in the teacher's note above.

GUIDING THEM OUT

When you're done, slowly rise to tabletop position on all fours, then guide your hips to your heels, bending your knees *(child's pose)*.

If it's comfortable for you, rest your hips on your heels and stretch your arms straight out in front of you, draping your chest to the floor.

Notice any resonant sensations you feel after practicing this boat breath. What quality describes your state of being now?

UJJAYI BREATH/ A.K.A. OCEAN BREATH

Time: 3-10 minutes (or longer, such as throughout an entire yoga practice ;)

Teacher's Note:

If you're a yoga teacher, you've probably practiced this breath quite a bit. Students tend to focus on the sound of the exhale, so breaking it down in this way allows them to figure out how to create the same quality and sound on the inhale as well.

It serves as a mental and physical anchor throughout vinyasa flow style yoga classes, helping students maintain their connection between body and mind as they focus their attention. You can also use this as a breathwork practice (outside of a yoga class).

Funny story, I was once almost in a four-car pile up in the fast lane of the freeway. I avoided the accident by a hair, and I noticed that I'd automatically shifted into ujjayi breath. I'd trained it so well in my yoga practice, that my body knew instantly what to do to calm itself down in a challenging situation! So cool!

The Script:

This breathing technique is excellent for calming your nervous system, focusing your attention, and creating internal heat.

Ujjayi breath is best done while seated, so find a block or a pillow to place underneath your sitting bones if you'd like to use one.

We'll begin with a tall spine, chest lifted, and shoulders relaxed.

For this style of breathing, we generate a sound at the back of our throat that sounds like an ocean wave.

Some call it Darth Vadar breath because it sounds like the character from Star Wars.

Before we practice the complete breath, we'll break it down into simpler components. It can take some time to figure out, so be gentle and patient with yourself if you're just learning this style.

We'll be using diaphragmatic breaths throughout the practice.

Upon each and every inhale, allow your belly to expand, and at the end of each exhale, draw your ribs gently down and in.

Begin by inhaling through your nose, then exhaling through your mouth, making a "haaaaaa" sound. Twice more, inhale through your nose, exhale through your mouth, "haaaaaa".

Again.

Inhale nose, exhale, "haaaaaa".

Now we'll reverse that.

Open your mouth and make an "aaaaah" sound while you are inhaling. It's like the sound you'd make if you were surprised in slow motion.

Exhale, seal your lips and send the air out through your nose.

Inhale with your mouth open, "aaaaah" sound.

Exhale, breathing out through your nose.

Last time like this, inhale mouth open, with sound, exhale mouth closed.

Okay, we're ready for the full Ujjayi Breath now. You'll keep your lips sealed on both your inhale and your exhale, breathing in and out of your nose only.

Let's do it.

Inhale, create a little hug at the back of your throat as you make the "haaaaa" sound.

Exhale, keep the slight contraction at the back of your throat - same sound, same quality.

Again, keep your lips sealed, inhale, and create an ocean sound at the back of your throat.

 Exhale, same sound.

Once more, inhale slowly and deeply.

Exhale completely.

Continue the ocean-sounding breath with lips sealed for the next _____ minutes. *(As long as you've allotted for breathwork today, or if teaching a vinyasa flow style yoga class, invite students to utilize this breath throughout their entire practice until they rest at the end in savasana.)*

PRANA & APANA

Time: Anywhere from 3-20 minutes

Teacher's Note:

This breathing practice offers an interplay between the upward flow of energy and the downward, grounding flow, making it an ideal complement to themes of balance, polarity, or yin/yang.

In this practice, we'll be utilizing mula bandha, or the pelvic floor lock. If you plan to guide students in mula bandha during your yoga teaching, it would be beneficial to introduce this breath at the beginning of the class. This way, students will know how to engage it when you cue it during class.

The Script:

This breath is best practiced while seated with a tall spine.

Feel free to place a yoga block, pillow, or cushion underneath you for support.

Prana is our life force, the energy most associated with inhaling. It generates a light, uplifting, expanding feeling.

Apana is downward, rooting energy, which provides grounding and calming sensations.

To connect more fully with the stabilizing energy at the base of your torso, we'll be employing mula bandha, our root lock, drawing our pelvic floors in and up.

Let's try that now, engaging the muscles there, drawing them in and up.

And release.

As we play with these two energies, a sublime dance of free-flowing energy occurs.

We'll also be visualizing color as we breathe.

For some, this comes easily, whereas others may find it challenging.

If you are in the latter camp, imagine what it would be like watching a sci-fi movie of yourself with CGI as you practice this breathing technique.

Let's begin.

Inhale, and draw an imaginary electric blue line of energy from the root of your torso, (your pelvic floor), up into your chest.

Take a pause, and allow the color to disappear.

Exhale, imagine a bright red light that begins at your chest and travels straight down to your pelvic floor.

At the end of your exhale, lift your pelvic floor up *(Mula Bandha)*.

Take a pause, and allow the color to disappear.

Relax your pelvic floor, and inhale, imagine the blue light traveling from the base of your torso up into your chest. Pause. The blue light disappears.

Exhale imagine a red light that moves from your chest down to your pelvic floor.

At the end of your exhale, engage your pelvic floor muscles and pause.

The red light disappears.

Continue.

Inhale, and guide the blue light from the base of your torso up to your chest.

Pause, hold.

Exhale, guide the red light from your chest down back down, engaging your pelvic floor.

Keep going on your own...

Notice how the inhale and the blue light generates a light, expansive, lifting feeling. Observe how the exhale and the red light provides a grounding, secure, stabilizing feeling.

Continue to breathe in this way for the next ____ minutes.
(The time you've allotted)

Release breath control and allow your breath to normalize.

(Wait for about 20 seconds)

How do you feel after utilizing your breath and alternating energies in this way?

(Wait for about 20 seconds)

There is no right or wrong answer. There is only inquiry and awareness.

ROOT & HEART CHAKRA BREATH

Time: Anywhere from 3-20 minutes

Teacher's Note:
This breathing pattern is very similar to the Prana & Apana breath above, except that we're bringing in the concept of the chakras and changing the colors to those that correlate with the chakras. It can be used around Valentine's Day, or with any themes around building a sense of safety and security within one's self and/or opening the heart or heart opening poses if you're focusing on those within your yoga class.

The Script:
This breath is best practiced while seated with a tall spine.

Feel free to place a yoga block, pillow, or cushion underneath your hips for support.

Lift your chest, and allow your shoulder blades to waterfall down your back.

We'll be focusing on our root chakra, located at the base of our torso, associated with safety and security, as well as our heart chakra, located in the center of our breastbone, associated with giving and receiving love freely.

We'll also be engaging our mula bandha, the muscles at the center of the perineum (the base of our pelvic floor). Engaging mula bandha has the effect of retaining energy, as well as establishing a sense of calmness and stabilization.

When we feel safe and secure, it's easier to maintain an open, loving heart.

We'll also be visualizing color.

For some, this comes easily, whereas others may find it challenging.

If you are in the latter camp, imagine what it would be like watching a sci-fi movie of yourself with CGI as you practice this breathing technique.

Let's begin.

Guide your awareness to the base of your torso, your root chakra.

Imagine a sphere of energy there, the color red.

Exhale, focus there, engaging your pelvic floor by lifting the muscles up.

Soften the muscular engagement now and inhale, draw a line of energy from your root, up into your chest, envisioning an emerald green orb there, your heart chakra.

Retain your breath. Feel your chest warm and expand.

Exhale, and imagine the line of energy traveling back down to your pelvic floor, the color red.

At the end of your exhale, engage your pelvic floor (mula bandha).

Pause, safe and secure.

Relax your pelvic floor, and inhale, imagine the line of energy traveling from the base of your torso up into your heart chakra.

 Brilliant green.

Hold your breath. Open chest, open-hearted.

Exhale, and imagine the energy moving from your chest down to your pelvic floor, back to the color red.

At the end of your exhale, engage your pelvic floor muscles and pause.

Continue. Inhale, guide the line of energy from the base of your torso up into your heart center, brilliant green, warm and expansive.

Retain.

Exhale, guide the line of energy from your chest down back down, engaging your pelvic floor. Tuning in to the color red, stable and secure.

Keep going on your own...

Notice how the inhale and tuning into your heart chakra generates a warm, expansive, lifting feeling. Observe how the exhale and focusing on your root chakra provides a grounding, secure, stabilizing feeling.

Continue to breathe in this way for the next ___minutes.
(*The time you've allotted*).

Release breath control and allow your breath to normalize.

(*Wait about 20 seconds.*)

As you assimilate the sensations from utilizing your breath and alternating energies in this way, what is the general feeling that you are experiencing now?

(*Wait about 20 seconds.*)

There is no right or wrong answer. There is only inquiry and awareness.

GUIDING THEM OUT

Food for thought:

The trust that you place in people outside of you that allows you to feel secure is transitory because attention and love can change or be withdrawn.

Instead, recognize that you can experience everlasting security based on the knowledge that you are a child of the universe, a fractal of source, and because of that you are always 100% lovable, worthy, and inherently belong.

Trust yourself to discern which situations and relationships are right for you and you will experience the innate security that allows you not only to give and receive love, but to BE LOVE.

When you do this, you will no longer be grasping and clinging to others, wanting them to behave in a certain way so that you can feel safe.

You will be open, confident, and relaxed, as you live with an open heart, both giving and receiving love with ease.

FIGURE 8 BREATH FOR BUILDING ENERGY

Time: 5-10 minutes

Teacher's Note:
This breath is excellent for practicing focused visualization by directing attention and attuning the mind to guide energy along the body's central line. It typically induces an uplifting, energetic shift, making it more suitable for the beginning of a yoga class rather than just before savasana. When incorporating this breath into a retreat, workshop, or meditation class, consider the most appropriate time for the heightened response it tends to elicit.

The Script:
This breathing technique is wonderful for training your point of focus and releasing stagnations by moving energy through your system.

It's best practiced while in a seated posture, with your spine erect. Feel free to sit on a pillow, meditation cushion, bolster, or yoga block for support.

It includes visualization as well as breathing. If you find it challenging to visualize, just pretend that you're watching a movie of yourself with computer-generated imagery (CGI) and imagine what it would look like.

We'll be making a neon-blue figure 8 from the base of the torso to the crown of the head, with the intersection point at the lower neck.

It's a little bit tricky, but if you try it a few times,
you'll get the hang of it.

Begin by imagining a bright, neon blue light at the base of your torso.

As you guide this light along with your breath, imagine it activating and energizing every place it touches along the way.

Slowly inhale as you draw the light up the front of your body, over your collar bone, crossing through to the back of your neck, up the back of your head to your crown.

Slowly exhale as you draw the brilliant blue light down your forehead, nose, and chin, crossing through your neck down your spine to the base of your torso.

Again. Inhale, guide the blue light from the base of your torso up the front of your body, crossing through your lower neck, up the back of your head to your crown.

Exhale, draw the light down your forehead, nose, and chin, crossing through at your neck, down the back of your spine to the root of your body.

One more time with me guiding. Slowly inhale as the blue light moves from the root of your torso up the front of your body, through your neck, up the back of your head to your crown.

Slow exhale as the blue, neon light moves down the front of your face, crossing through your neck, down your spine, and back to the root of your body.

Continue this breathing pattern and the Figure 8 visualization for the next ___ minutes. *(as much time as you've allotted for breathing today)*

Release the visualization and begin to normalize your breath.

Sit for a bit longer as you stabilize.

You may notice that your mind feels more clear and alert, and your body feels revitalized and energetic after cycling your breath and energy this way.

Check-in and see if this is the case.

What effect did this type of breath have on your system today?

ALTERNATE NOSTRIL BREATH WITH RETENTION & 3RD EYE ACTIVATION

Time: 5-10 minutes

Teacher's Note:

Neuroscientists such as Dr. Jeffrey Fannin have found that when we're in a state of stress our brain activity localizes in either one hemisphere or the other.

If we are overly emotional, the right side.

If we're over-analyzing, spinning out, the left side.

Whole brain activities, such as Alternate Nostril Breath create hemispheric integration and communication, turning on both hemispheres, resulting in a brain balance, providing access to enhanced information and greater equanimity.

Alternate Nostril Breath is mentioned in the following texts: Hatha Yoga Pradipika, Gheranda Samhita, Tirumandiram, Siva Samhita, Puranas, and in the Upanishads. Some suggest ending the breath practice by exhaling through the left nostril, as this has the most calming, cooling effect on the system.

You can choose to guide each and every breath, or you may wish to guide a few rounds as I've scripted here and then allow practitioners to continue on their own for a specified amount of time.

The Script:

This type of breath increases oxygen flow and drives communication between both the left and right hemispheres of your brain, promoting clarity and calmness while diminishing stress and anxiety.

It is best done seated with your spine tall and chest lifted. If you'd like support, sit on a pillow, bolster, yoga block, or meditation cushion.

Using your right hand, place your index and middle finger between your eyebrows.

We're adding this little bonus effect with finger placement here, as it lines up directly with your pineal gland, the seat of your intuition, and the gateway into higher consciousness.

First, take a deep breath in, and exhale all of your breath out.

Now cover your right nostril with your thumb, and inhale through the left nostril.

Gently seal your left nostril with your third finger, retain your breath, and hold (*about 2-3 full seconds is the amount for each breath-hold*).

Release your right thumb and exhale through your right nostril.

Inhale, right side.

Place your thumb over the right nostril again, and retain your breath.

Release your third finger and exhale through the left side.

This is one full round.

Again. Inhale, left side, seal, and retain.
Exhale right.

Inhale right, seal, and retain.
Exhale left.

Inhale left nostril, retain.
Exhale right.

Inhale right side, retain.
Exhale Left.

Continue for as long as you have allotted for this breath practice. If you are teaching this practice to others, you may choose to continue to guide each breath, or you can have the students continue on their own.

Release the alternate nostril breath *(ending the cycle by exhaling out of the left nostril if you'd like to follow the yogic texts.),* allowing your hands to rest on your thighs.

Sit up nice and tall.

Allow your breath to normalize.

Now that you've balanced the logical, left hemisphere of your brain with the emotional, creative, right hemisphere, you may find yourself in a more relaxed, even state.

You have access to more creative solutions with enhanced awareness, and with the third eye connection, a reminder to listen to your intuition and inner knowing.

DIRGHA BREATH/ 3-PART BREATH (Short Practice)

Time: 3-10 minutes

Teacher's Note:

When we're in a state of dysregulation and stress, we tend to take shallow, shorter, and more frequent breaths.

By consciously expanding our stomachs outward, we draw our diaphragms down, creating space in the thoracic cavity and allowing access to the full capacity of our lungs.

This enables our breath to flow easily and without restriction. Engaging in slow, conscious, diaphragmatic breaths sends a signal to our nervous system that we're safe and everything is alright.

This practice delivers maximum oxygen and improves various processes in our body.

The Script:

Shallow breathing can lower oxygenation, decrease immune function, and increase our body's stress response.

This breathing technique comes to the rescue by encouraging greater oxygen exchange and can lower our heart rate, stabilize our blood pressure, and calm our nervous system.

For this practice, you'll be seated.

Feel free to sit on a folded-up blanket, bolster, or meditation pillow for support. Lengthen your spine, and rest your palms downward facing on your thighs.

Inhale, fill up your lower belly, midsection, then upper chest.

Exhale, release the air from your upper chest, midsection, then lower belly.

Repeat this again.

Inhale, fill up your belly, then your midsection and upper chest. Exhale, release... upper, middle, lower.

Now bring your awareness to the back of your body.

Inhale, and fill up your low, middle, and upper back.

Exhale, release the air from your upper, middle, then lower back.

Repeat.

Inhale, fill up your low, middle, and upper back.

Exhale, release the air from your upper, middle, then lower back.

Now both front and back at the same time.

In fact, more than that - a three-dimensional breath, utilizing the entire 360-degree circumference of your torso.

Inhale, expand your lower torso, midsection, then entire upper body,

and exhale, release the air from your upper, middle, then lower sections.

Again, fill up your lower, middle, and upper body, and exhale, release the air from the upper, middle, then low section.

Continue this three-dimensional, three-part breath for the
next ___minutes. *(The remaining time allotted).*

If your mind wanders, without judgment, just simply guide your
awareness back to your breath.

DIRGHA BREATH/ 3-PART BREATH (Long Practice)

Time: Anywhere from 5-20 minutes

Teacher's Note:

In this longer 3-Part Breath practice, practitioners use their hands as a tactile guide for better diaphragm engagement.

It's a helpful way to ensure the diaphragm is working effectively and at the right pace, allowing the concept to sink in while maximizing oxygen intake.

The Script:

This breathing practice encourages higher levels of oxygenation by training the use of your entire lung capacity. The full, deep, diaphragmatic breaths will also help you de-stress by calming and relaxing your nervous system.

You can practice this breath on your back or seated. If sitting, feel free to sit on a yoga block or cushion for support.

Lift your chest and lengthen your spine.

Place your hands on your lower belly.

Inhale, and fill up your lower belly like a balloon.
Exhale, feel your belly soften down and in.

Inhale, expand your lower belly into your hands, and exhale, feel your lower belly fall.

Continue for three more rounds.

Next, place your hands on your rib cage as if you are wearing your hands like a second set of ribs.

Keep a couple of inches of space in between your middle fingers.

Inhale, expand your ribs outwards,
pressing your hands out with the power of your breath, and
exhale draw your ribs down and in.

Think Superman or Superwoman, with a big barrel chest.

Inhale, expand your ribs out sideways.
Exhale, ribs come down and in.

Continue this for three more rounds.

Now bring your hands to your upper chest so that your index fingers
touch your collarbone and your elbows point downwards.

Inhale, fill up your low belly, midsection, then upper chest, feeling
your hands rise as you send the breath there.

Exhale, release the air from your upper chest, midsection, then lower
belly.

Inhale, low, middle, upper chest, hands lifted by your breath.
Exhale, release the air from your upper, middle, then lower belly.

Continue this for three more rounds.

Relax your arms down by your sides, and continue the three-part
breath for the next ___minutes. *(The remaining time you've allotted for
this practice).*

If you find your mind drifting onto something else, no worries or
guilt, just come back to guiding your breath again.

OBSTACLE REMOVING BREATH

Time: 10-15 minutes

Teacher's Note:
This breathing practice utilizes the breath as a vehicle for inner transformation, enabling practitioners to discover and release any present blockages while welcoming qualities that can provide the greatest support in their current lives. As the breath moves and flows, answers may more naturally arise, and we can use the power of breath to bring about positive changes.

P.S. This one's pretty heady, more like a guided inner inquiry assisted by the breath. Allow some time for reflection when practitioners are asked to bring to mind an answer, otherwise, it will start to feel too jumbled.

Just take your time and pace it out.

The Script:
This breathing technique helps you clear the blockages from your path as you strengthen your inner resolve and draw in qualities that support you.

For this breathing practice, feel free to lie down on your back or sit up tall. If on your back, you may wish to place a pillow or bolster under your knees. If seated, feel free to place a block or bolster under your hips for support.

Close your eyes and take a few deep, relaxed breaths. Consider one goal that you have for yourself or for your life right now. It can be anything you want. A quality you wish to cultivate, something you want to create or achieve, or even having a better relationship with someone. The sky's the limit.

(Allow some time here to consider...)

Take a slow, deep, diaphragmatic breath through your nose for a count of 6, 5, 4, 3, 2, 1,

and exhale it out through your nose for 6, 5, 4, 3, 2, 1.

Inhale fill up your belly, 6, 5, 4, 3, 2, 1,
and exhale, belly softens, 6, 5, 4, 3, 2, 1.

Adding a hold,

Inhale 6, 5, 4, 3, 2, 1.
Hold - 4, 3, 2, 1.

Exhale 6, 5, 4, 3, 2, 1.
Hold - 4, 3, 2, 1.

Inhale 6, 5, 4, 3, 2, 1.
Longer hold 5, 4, 3, 2, 1.

Exhale 6, 5, 4, 3, 2, 1.
Hold 5, 4, 3, 2, 1,

Slowly inhale, nice and easy, and allow your breath to return to normal, releasing the breath control.

Consider one internal thing that could be blocking you from your goal. Something like fear, self-doubt, or discouragement.

Ensure that it's also only one or two words in length.

When you consider this thing, how does it feel in your body? Where do you notice it the most?

(Pause here to allow time to figure out how and where it's felt.)

Now bring to mind one quality that would support your goal, like strength, determination, healthy cells, or patience.

Make sure that it's one word or two words at the most.

When you bring up this quality, how does it feel in your body?

(Pause here to allow time to figure out how and where it's felt.)

Now take a slow, deep, belly breath.

As you inhale, fill up with the positive, supportive quality you selected and all the sensations that come with it.

As you exhale, release the negative, limiting one and its corresponding feelings along with your breath.

Stay with these two words and the associated feelings they inspire for 3 more breaths.

Inhale, slowly fill up with the empowering quality, and exhale slowly, releasing the limitation.

Same again. Inhale, fill up with this powerful quality, exhale, and release the obstacle.

Take one more breath just like that.

Inhale the helpful feeling, and exhale letting go of everything else.

Return to your regular breath.

Let's dig a little deeper this time and look beneath the surface of the previous two.

Identify something that may have been previously hidden from your awareness, but in this state of presence is available to you now.

Within your being, what else is blocking you from this goal?
(pause)...And what is underneath that?... Feeling unworthy?

Unlovable? Something else?

When you think of this thing, how does it show up in your body?

Where do you feel it? What does it feel like?

(Pause here to allow time to figure out how and where it's felt.)

Now we need something even more powerful to put in its place.

Identify one more internal quality that is needed to support you in your endeavor.

Love, self-worth, acceptance, or something else?

When you consider this powerful, high-vibrational quality, how does it feel within you?

Where do you feel it?

(Pause here, to allow time to figure out how and where it's felt.)

Now take a slow, deep inhale, filling up with this high-vibrational attribute, and slowly exhale, releasing the underlying blockage that was holding you back.

Again, slowly Inhale this supportive quality and all of the expansive feelings it brings along with it, and slowly exhale releasing the dense one along with all of its associated gunk.

Last time.

Inhale, fill all the way up with the expansive, high-vibrational quality, and exhale every last bit of the blockage out.

Allow your breath to return to normal.

Let the fluctuations of your mind settle into stillness.

(Wait about 30 seconds.)

GUIDING THEM OUT

Now that you are in a more expansive, clear state of being, ask yourself if you feel called to take any action step in your life right now - a playful exploration of the potential you just created.

Wait and see if you receive an answer.

Feel free to enjoy silence for a few more minutes.

When you are ready to complete your meditation, slowly open your eyes.

If you received guidance to do an action step, follow up with it as soon as possible.

SUN BREATH - ENERGY FIELD AMPLIFIER

Time: 4-10 minutes

Teacher's Note:
Sun Breath provides a simple method to fortify the energy of one's auric field, making it especially valuable for those who are more apt to take on the energy and emotions of others.

It amplifies divine inner power and is especially beneficial to use when energy feels depleted, unstable, or prior to entering crowded environments or events where there may be an overwhelming amount of different types of energy.

The Script:
Rather than shielding or protecting your energy, this breath strengthens and stabilizes your energy field.

Consider the analogy of a child on the playground: one with low self-esteem becomes a target for bullies and may feel overwhelmed by the energy of others. In contrast, a confident and self-assured child isn't an energetic match for this.

Through this breathwork, our energy field becomes fortified and stable, revitalizing our energy and reducing the likelihood of taking on other people's stuff.

Let's begin.

Sit up tall, and feel free to sit on a bolster for support.

Call to mind a memory of the most unconditional love you have ever experienced in your life. It may be the love you received from a parent, relative, friend, lover, teacher/coach, or your pet (dog, cat).

Localize this feeling of love at the very center of your chest (your heart chakra center).

Embed the feeling within a bright golden light there, about the size of a golf ball.

You'll be utilizing diaphragmatic breaths, expanding your stomach, ribs, and chest as you inhale, and softening your rib cage as you exhale, letting out your breath evenly and slowly.

Your lips are sealed on both your inhale and your exhale, breathing through your nose.

Inhale, allow the golden light to grow a few inches bigger.
Exhale, strengthen the energy.

Inhale, fill your chest and upper back with bright golden light.
Exhale, strengthen the energy.

Inhale, expand the energy to fill your entire torso,
Exhale, fortify the energy.

Inhale expanding the golden light throughout your entire body,
your legs, your arms, your head.
Exhale, feel your entire auric field strengthening.

Any imbalanced, weakened, or darkened spots resuming
full vibrant health.

Inhale, radiate the golden light out beyond your body,
about five or six feet in all directions.

Exhale, feel this entire area stabilizing,
buzzing with well-being and radiance.

Notice how you feel now.

Experiencing your own energy from the inside extending out like the sun's rays.

(If doing a longer meditation read this sentence and then pause for two minutes.) Stay here for a couple more minutes, maintaining your connection to these sensations as you continue to breathe in and out of your nose with full deep breaths.

GUIDING THEM OUT

Begin to bring your awareness back.

Allow your breath to normalize.

As you go out into the world, you will be more apt to notice when you feel something that doesn't belong to you.

It's important to remind yourself that you don't need to take on other peoples' thoughts, emotions, or energy as your own.

When you're balanced within your own energy field, you may find that you feel better throughout the day, and you may enjoy social situations a whole lot more.

INCREASE YOUR ENERGY FIELD 6 - 3 - 6 - 3 BREATH

Time: 5 - 20 minutes

Teacher's Note:

Here's another breathing practice that strengthens our personal energy field, providing a sense of inner stability and vibrance.

Within a Pranic Healing Course that I took at the California Institute for Human Science, we did an experiment where we measured the energy fields of all students prior to this breath and afterwards.

We discovered that each of us experienced an increase in the measurement of the auric/energy field surrounding the body after only a few minutes of this breath.

After guiding practitioners through the few rounds that are scripted below, you may continue to guide each breath, or have them continue on their own.

The Script:

This breathwork practice helps us connect to our energy field, enhancing its strength in a way that allows us to feel centered and stable.

When our auric field is increased, we are less susceptible to being overcome by the emotions and energy of other people and places, and can eliminate the need to "shield" ourselves because we're fortified from the inside out.

This breath is best practiced while seated.

Find a comfortable position, and feel free to place a pillow, bolster, or cushion underneath you for support.

Lift your chest and relax your shoulders.

The breathing pattern is rhythmic, with the inhale and exhale exactly twice as long as the pause in between which helps put the mind in a trance-like state.

For this breath, you will inhale for a count of six, retain your breath for a count of three, exhale for a count of six, then hold empty for a count of three.

Use your diaphragm, inflating your belly on your inhalation, and deflating it on your exhalation.

Breathe in and out of your nose only, keeping your lips sealed.

You may enhance the experience by imagining your body glowing.... any color that you choose: gold, silver, iridescent, or any other color that you choose.

As you continue to breathe in this style, imagine your energy glowing more and more vibrantly and expanding in all directions around your body.

Let's begin.

Inhale, 6, 5, 4, 3, 2, 1.
Hold your breath for 3, 2, 1.

Exhale, 6, 5, 4, 3, 2, 1.
Hold empty for 3, 2, 1.

Again,

Inhale, 6, 5, 4, 3, 2, 1.
Hold your breath for 3, 2, 1.

Exhale, 6, 5, 4, 3, 2, 1.
Hold empty, 3, 2, 1.

Feeling the rhythm...

Inhale, 6, 5, 4, 3, 2, 1.
Hold your breath 3, 2, 1.

Exhale, 6, 5, 4, 3, 2, 1.
Hold empty 3, 2, 1.

Inhale, 6, 5, 4, 3, 2, 1.
Hold, 3, 2, 1.

Exhale, 6, 5, 4, 3, 2, 1.
Hold empty, 3, 2, 1.

Continue for the next ___ minutes.
(However long you've allotted for this breathwork today)

GUIDING THEM OUT

Begin to normalize your breath.

Take a pause, finding stillness within your mind.

Notice how you feel and how your energy feels.

Feel free to utilize this breath anytime you want to calm your mind and emotions, promote vitality and renewal, and stabilize your state of being.

BREATHING TO INCREASE PERSONAL POWER /
6 - 3 - 9 - 6 BREATH

Time: about 10 minutes but can continue for a few more minutes if you like.

Teacher's note:
This breathing practice employs a long exhale to relax the nervous system and engagement of uddiyana bandha to connect to the strength at one's center.

For yoga instructors, it would be great to have students practice this if you're theming around personal power or inner strength, and/or before vinyasa or power yoga classes so that they can connect to their core.

For meditation instructors and wellness practitioners, use this anytime you'd like to help people experience a state of calm, confident presence.

The Script:
So many of us look outside of ourselves for a sense of safety and stability.

Waiting for conditions to be a certain way so that we can feel a certain way.

Since outside conditions are transitory, we can never find the sense of safety and assurance that we're looking for.

It has to come from within.

When we trust ourselves and feel safe and steady within ourselves, we take these qualities with us wherever we go, feeling more confident and comfortable in all situations and places.

This breathing practice helps you connect to your sense of calm, inner strength, and personal power.

There is a longer exhale which calms your nervous system, and at the end of the exhale, a connection to the power center behind your navel.

This place at the center of your abdomen and organs has been recognized by yogis, Qi Gong practitioners, meditators, martial artists, and fitness professionals as a place of mastery, strength, wisdom, and tranquility. It is your physical and energetic core.

This breath practice is best done seated with a tall spine.

Feel free to sit on a bolster for support.

You'll be utilizing diaphragmatic breaths, expanding your stomach, ribs, and chest as you inhale, and softening your rib cage as you inhale, letting out your breath evenly and slowly.

When you inhale, notice the expansion of your belly, midsection, then upper body.

You'll pause for a short breath retention, which has an uplifting energizing mental effect.

Then you'll exhale slowly, and at the end of your exhale, you'll draw your navel gently back towards your spine.

With this mild contraction at your navel, connect to the power at your center with awareness.

We'll begin with a six-count, then we'll add on.

Inhale for a count of 6, 5, 4, 3, 2, 1.
Exhale for a count of 6, 5, 4, 3, 2, 1.

Again, inhale for 6, 5, 4, 3, 2, 1.
Exhale for 6, 5, 4, 3, 2, 1.

Adding breath retention...

(Speaking slowly for the six-count inhale)
Inhale, fill up your belly, midsection, and then your chest.

Hold your breath for 3, 2, 1.

(Speaking slowly for the six-count exhale)
Exhale, release the air from your chest, midsection, then belly.

(Speaking slowly for the six-count hold)
Hold, draw your navel towards your spine, and feel the presence of your personal power

(Speaking for this six-count inhale)
Again, inhale fill-up from the bottom to the top of your lungs.

Hold your breath for 3, 2, 1.

Exhale fully for 6, 5, 4, 3, 2, 1.

And hold empty for 6, 5, 4, 3, 2, 1.

Adding a longer exhale now....

Inhale for 6, 5, 4, 3, 2, 1.

Hold your breath for 3, 2, 1.

Exhale for 9, 8, 7, 6, 5, 4, 3, 2, 1.

(Say these words instead of the six-count)
At the end of your exhale, hold, and gently draw your navel towards your spine. Notice the stabilizing, empowering effect.

Inhale for 6, 5, 4, 3, 2, 1.

Hold your breath for 3, 2, 1.

Exhale for 9, 8, 7, 6, 5, 4, 3, 2, 1.

And hold 6, 5, 4, 3, 2, 1.

Again, inhale for 6, 5, 4, 3, 2, 1.

Hold your breath for 3, 2, 1.

Exhale for 9, 8, 7, 6, 5, 4, 3, 2, 1.

(Say these words instead of the six-count)
Hold, navel to spine, feeling your energy gather and fortify.

Inhale, 6, 5, 4, 3, 2, 1.

Hold your breath for 3, 2, 1.

Exhale, 9, 8, 7, 6, 5, 4, 3, 2, 1.

(Say these words instead of the six-count)
Hold empty; navel gently to spine, steady and centered.

Continue the 6 - 3 - 9 - 6 breathing pattern for the next ___minutes.
(As long as you've allotted for breathwork today)

GUIDING THEM OUT

Allow your breath to slowly return to normal now.

When you've completed the practice, notice the after-effects.

What is the general state of your mind?

How does your body feel?

Is any emotion or quality present?

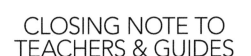

CLOSING NOTE TO TEACHERS & GUIDES

I hope that you found this resource valuable. It was my wish to share more than 15 years of compiled resources with you to make your life easier and to help your students expand and evolve in all ways.

I hope the ideas inside have evolved for you as well, with your own spin, voice, and perspective. Maybe you will be inspired to leave the next generation of yoga, meditation, and wellness guides with your own discoveries, learnings, and resources.

If you want to dive deeper into consciousness awakening and best operating practices for this amazing bodymindspirit head over to radicalenlightenment.com.

We have a complimentary Choose-Your-Place-In-Nature Personalized Transformation Meditation for you there.

With so much love,

Kelli

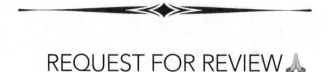

REQUEST FOR REVIEW 🙏

Dear Yoga, Meditation, and Wellness Community,

Your journey with this book, filled with meditation scripts, inspirations, and breathwork practices, has the power to help other people awaken, enliven, and heal.

If you've found value in its pages,
please leave a brief review on Amazon by going to www.soulfulscripts/review.

Your review matters because it can make the book more visible to others, illuminating the path for fellow teachers, students, and seekers.

For our shared goal of helping others experience greater inner peace, freedom, and transformation, please take a moment to post your review on my Amazon page and be a guiding light for those seeking wisdom and well-being.

With heartfelt gratitude,
Kelli

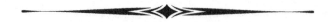

ABOUT THE AUTHOR

Kelli Russell is a seasoned wellness guide, with the highest yoga teacher trainer credentials offered through Yoga Alliance (500-ERYT + YACEP). She's taught yoga and meditation for studios, private clients, and corporations since 2009, and founded YogaBoost, a pioneering corporate yoga company designed to counteract the adverse impact of modern sedentary lifestyles.

With a degree in Psychology and a Master's in Counseling, Kelli combines her understanding of the human psyche with her expertise in yoga and spirituality to facilitate deep personal transformations that align people with their true selves.

In 2015, her journey took an intriguing turn when she witnessed the incredible healing of her best friend's back pain through emotional kinesiology, inspiring her to embark on a path of training in Psychological Kinesiology and Emotional Energy Healing. Now, as a Subconscious Change Facilitator, Kelli offers individual sessions both internationally via Zoom and in person in Encinitas, CA to help people release stress, anxiety, and past trauma, and establish positive subconscious beliefs so that they can meet their goals and embrace life with confidence, clarity, and inner freedom.

Kelli is deeply committed to sharing her resources with fellow yoga teachers, wellness practitioners, and spiritual guides, as the collective power of awakening, enlivening, and healing contributes to greater global harmony, enhancing the quality of life for all.

To explore the realm of Subconscious Change, visit www.rapidtransformationsessions.com.